YOU AND YOUR PREMATURE BABY

BARBARA GLOVER is a primary school teacher, and the mother of a premature baby.

CHRISTINE HODSON is an SRN and midwife, with experience of working in Special Care Baby Units. She was trained at Leeds Maternity Hospital.

HEALTHCARE FOR WOMEN SERIES

Coping with Stress
Georgia Witkin-Lanoil

Eating Well for a Healthy Pregnancy
Dr Barbara Pickard

Everything You Need to Know about the Pill
Wendy Cooper and Dr Tom Smith

How to Get Pregnant & How Not To
P. Bello, Dr C. Dolto and Dr A. Schiffmann

Lifting the Curse: How to relieve painful periods
Beryl Kingston

Menopause: A practical, self-help guide for women
Raewyn Mackenzie

Successful Breastfeeding
Joan Neilson

Taking Care of Your Skin
Dr Vernon Coleman

Thrush: How it's caused and what to do about it
Caroline Clayton

Women and Depression: A practical self-help guide
Deidre Sanders

Women and Tranquillisers
Celia Haddon

Women's Problems: An A to Z
Dr Vernon Coleman

You and Your Caesarean Birth
Trisha Duffett-Smith

You and Your Premature Baby
Barbara Glover and Christine Hodson

HEALTHCARE FOR WOMEN

YOU AND YOUR PREMATURE BABY

Barbara Glover and Christine Hodson, SRN, SCM

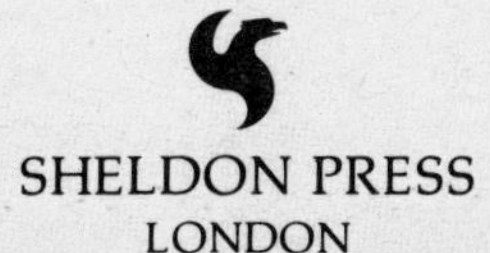

SHELDON PRESS
LONDON

First published in Great Britain in 1985 by
Sheldon Press, SPCK, Marylebone Road, London NW1 4DU

Thanks are due to W. H. Freeman and Company for permission to quote extracts from *Born Too Soon* by S. Goldberg and B. DiVitto. Copyright © 1983.

British Library Cataloguing in Publication Data

Glover, Barbara
You and your premature baby.—(Healthcare for women)
1. Infants (Premature)
I. Title II. Hodson, Christine III. Series
618.92'011'0240431 RJ250

ISBN 0-85969-475-5
ISBN 0-85969-476-3 Pbk

Typeset by Photobooks (Bristol) Ltd.
Printed in Great Britain by
Richard Clay (The Chaucer Press) Ltd,
Bungay, Suffolk

Dedication

This book is dedicated to all the parents who shared their experiences with us. We were privileged to witness the quiet courage of ordinary families in their suffering and love for these precious babies.

Contents

Introduction

Over 40,000[1] babies are born alive each year in England weighing no more than 5½ lbs (2500 g). Of those, about 12,500 babies each weigh less than a couple of bags of sugar, and about 1500 are so tiny that they are lighter than a carton of fruit juice. Of all these small babies, 94 per cent survive, thanks to the magnificent dedication of our doctors and nurses, and the modern technological equipment in our hospitals. Most of these babies not only survive, but grow up to be healthy, happy, normal children. One of these is Tamsin Glover, Barbara's daughter, who was born nine weeks prematurely weighing only 3 lbs 4 oz (1470 g). At birth she suffered from pneumonia and a collapsed lung, and at three days old was baptized in her incubator by the hospital chaplain. She was expected to die. However, the medical staff at St Mary's Hospital, Manchester, and the Royal Lancaster Infirmary Special Care Baby Unit were determined that she should live. The Registrar at Lancaster worked immediately on her collapsed lung, and saved her life. Slowly she recovered, and today is a very lively, affectionate child, full of energy and happiness.

Tamsin spent the first month of her life in hospital, growing stronger and fitter week by week in preparation for that special day when at last she could join her family at home. During this month Barbara tried to find out as much as she could about premature, or preterm, babies.

> I wanted to learn everything I could about preterm babies, so that I could give Tamsin the best help possible. I scoured bookshops and libraries, but I was astonished to discover that there was nothing available. So we had to manage by ourselves. We shambled through the first months, often feeling frustrated and helpless. At around 4 lbs 2 oz (1870 g) she was too tiny for normal baby clothes—my best quality nappies were impossibly

huge. How can we get her to take all her tablets and medicine? Why does she cry so much? The problems seemed endless, but gradually we solved them for ourselves. Sometimes during the peace and stillness of the 2 a.m. feed I would think of all we had gone through, and I desperately wanted to share my new-found knowledge with new 'prem' mums. I wanted to help them cope with their tiny babies, and to solve the problems, practical and otherwise. In my gratitude for my own baby's life I wanted to lighten their load.

And so this book was born. Its purpose is to give parents of premature babies as much help, information, and advice as possible so that they have a better chance to cope with the trauma of an early birth.

Christine, a qualified midwife with experience of special care baby units, wrote the medical sections, and the result is a handbook of both medical information and practical help especially written for parents of preterm babies.

We hope that this book will give real help to the thousands of families who face the struggle to cope with the frightening and stressful experience of a baby born too soon.

As part of our research we appealed for help from parents of premature babies. We were delighted to receive over 250 letters and completed questionnaires, and we were able to use these experiences to support our findings. We have preserved the parents' and children's confidentiality by changing their names.

We would like to thank all those who gave us help and support in the production of this book, and especially Linda Blenkinship, Dr Trevor Matthews, *Good Housekeeping* magazine, the Lancaster branch of the National Childbirth Trust, and the Royal Lancaster Infirmary Special Care Baby Unit. Thanks to Pat Matthews who typed the manuscript, to Dr Bob Welch for giving us so much encouragement, and to our families for their help and understanding.

Throughout the text, babies are referred to as 'she' and doctors as 'he'. This is purely for grammatical convenience, and is not intended to be discriminatory in any way.

ONE

The Birth

> . . . the experience made me appreciate the psychological and emotional importance of the last weeks of a pregnancy. I had no time to prepare myself mentally for the baby's arrival.

For most parents, a premature delivery comes as a great shock. Psychological adjustment to the idea of a new baby takes place gradually over the full 40 weeks of a normal pregnancy. When the 40 weeks are abruptly cut short, many parents have great difficulty in accepting that the baby has arrived and the mother is no longer pregnant.

It is quite normal to feel cheated of pregnancy, cheated of the time you had planned ahead before the birth, and of course it is normal to search the preceding events for that elusive cause of premature labour.

In the first days after a premature delivery it is perfectly normal for the mother to blame herself. The important thing to remember is that preterm labour is *rarely caused by anything the mother has done during her pregnancy.* Of the 40,000 to 50,000 preterm babies born each year in this country, comparatively few premature births are actually explained and the cause seldom found.

Reasons for premature birth

Sudden onset of labour

A sudden onset of labour can occur anywhere at any time and to anyone. No one really understands the reasons why any labour starts, be it full-term or preterm. A sudden, unexpected onset of labour can take even the most placid person by surprise. A premature labour begins as does any full-term labour but it is all too easy to ignore the signs.

> I ignored my first signs of going into labour as I couldn't believe that it was possible at 32 weeks. It was a big shock to produce a premature baby.

Pre-eclampsia or pregnancy-induced hypertension

Pre-eclampsia or pregnancy-induced hypertension is one of several conditions that can occur during pregnancy making it necessary to induce or deliver the baby under emergency conditions in order to save mother and baby. A small proportion of preterm babies are born this way.

It occurs only during pregnancy and can be mild or severe in nature. The illness manifests itself as high blood pressure (hypertension), fluid retention causing swelling (called oedema) and protein in the urine (proteinuria).

When the blood pressure is high the amount of oxygen reaching the foetus via the placenta is diminished. Therefore development and growth may be impaired. If left undetected or untreated the danger is that the mother may have a type of fit, obviously putting herself and her baby at risk. This means that the baby has to be induced to arrive prematurely.

Bleeding in pregnancy

This is another emergency, although severe and profuse bleeding from the placenta is rare, and Caesarean section, performed to prevent bleeding, is a life-saving operation. Causes of bleeding may be:

- Placental abruption—when part of the placenta becomes detached from the wall of the uterus.

- Placenta praevia—when the placenta lies over the neck of the uterus it blocks baby's exit.

When the membranes rupture

Inside the uterus the baby is floating in amniotic fluid, enclosed within a warm secure world. Membranes form a tough bag or sac which normally breaks during labour. Occasionally the membranes rupture prematurely with no signs of labour and for no obvious reason. This causes the amniotic fluid to leak out via the mother's vagina. The risk of infection to the baby is greatly increased, and admission to hospital usually follows. If the mother gives extra attention to hygiene, is given antibiotics and bedrest, some doctors believe infection will not necessarily occur.

In the majority of mothers, labour will often start itself once the membranes have ruptured. The doctors may decide to induce labour if it is safe enough for the baby to be born. Sometimes the risk of staying inside the mother is greater than that of facing the outside world. When the waters break in early pregnancy every attempt to gain time, growth and development of the baby is usually given. It can be an anxious waiting time.

Multiple pregnancies

It is not expected that many mothers with a multiple pregnancy will carry their babies to full term of 40 weeks. This is thought to be due to the increased weight, pressure and possibly hormonal influence of the growing babies. It does appear to be policy to forewarn mothers carrying two or more babies that premature babies can be expected—of course every attempt to help the mother grow her babies for the maximum time is given. Hospital admission may be advised for rest at the crucial times of the pregnancy—usually between 28 and 32 weeks' gestation. In multiple births it is important to realize that *maturity* of the babies is far more relevant than the individual weights.

An irritable uterus

This is a condition in which the uterus becomes increasingly 'active' as the pregnancy progresses. In this condition preterm labour often starts and since the introduction of a drug called ritodrine (Yutopar), mothers with an irritable uterus have been helped to carry their babies to a reasonable gestation.

An abnormally shaped uterus

An abnormally shaped uterus can be detected by ultrasound scan, or can be seen during a Caesarean section. You may, or may not, be aware that your uterus has an abnormal shape. It can be the cause of problems during pregnancy, and it can lead to a premature labour.

An incompetent cervix
When the cervix is incompetent, the neck of the womb becomes slack and does not seem able to withstand the pressure of the growing foetus above it. The cervix opens up (as in labour) and a miscarriage occurs in the early weeks, or a premature baby in later weeks. This may be caused by hormones or by weak muscles in the cervix. Mothers who repeatedly miscarry pregnancies can be helped by the insertion of a stitch around the cervix. Occasionally, however, the labour still starts prematurely and the cervix begins to open up. The stitch must be removed by a doctor to avoid damage to the mother. Once the cervix starts to dilate labour has started and cannot be stopped.

Drugs to stop labour

Preterm labour can be stopped in some women with the use of drugs and rest, but it can always start again at any time in the pregnancy. The drug most commonly used is ritodrine (Yutopar). It can be given via a drip into the mother's arm or in tablet form and is used widely in maternity hospitals to help stop preterm labour.

Some 'difficult' pregnancies with several onsets of labour can be stopped and the baby helped to reach a reasonable maturity.

Lung maturity

The baby's lungs are bathed in a substance called surfactant which allows the many tiny air sacs in the lungs to expand allowing the exchange of oxygen and carbon dioxide. Surfactant starts to be produced at 22 weeks of pregnancy and in normal pregnancies a sharp increase occurs at 34 to 36 weeks. If surfactant is not present in a high enough quantity at the baby's birth breathing difficulties will occur.

Measurement of surfactant is of great value. Sometimes, if a premature labour seems imminent, a 24- to 48-hour course of a steroid is given by injection to the mother. This does seem to give a reduced risk of breathing difficulties in premature babies. It is thought the steroid stimulates the production of enzymes in the lungs to produce the surfactant.

Preparing yourself

Although the majority of the 40,000 to 50,000 premature babies born each year arrive quite unexpectedly—whether due to a sudden onset of labour or to an emergency—some mothers know that a preterm birth can be anticipated.

Preparation for a preterm birth is so important and of great value. The most important step to take if you know your baby will be premature is to visit the Special Care Baby Unit (SCBU). This will give you the opportunity to obtain a mental image of the unit, the staff, and to see some of the equipment that may be used to help your baby. Many maternity units do now include a brief visit to the SCBU during an antenatal tour of the unit. Ideally this visit should be before 24 weeks of pregnancy, but in many units it does seem, illogically, to be arranged during the last two months!

A few of the larger hospitals do now produce comprehensive booklets about their SCBU. Suggest a visit to the SCBU and hopefully the nurses will be only too willing to show you around. This can be a tremendous relief and prevent undue worrying.

Some antenatal wards provide parentcraft teaching for mothers who are in hospital for rest/observation during pregnancy. If you are missing clinic parentcraft and breathing/relaxation classes, ask for the sister to arrange these for you while you are in hospital. Preparation, both mental and practical, helps enormously.

Being in hospital antenatally for an indefinite length of time is not easy for you, your partner or your children. Take each day at a time. The baby will benefit from every extra day in the womb, so do rest and think positively. Take an interest in what will happen to your baby after birth, and how you can actively help.

It is routine to transfer mothers antenatally to another

larger hospital within the area, if a preterm baby is anticipated. The local maternity hospital may only have a small SCBU and it is possible the baby may require intensive care after birth. During labour the mother may benefit from the large back-up services only a larger hospital can give.

Labour

A preterm labour starts before 37 completed weeks of pregnancy. The premature baby is smaller than its full-term counterpart, but this does not necessarily mean that labour and delivery will be any the less painful, quicker or easier.

Ideally, preterm labours should be conducted within a hospital with specialist staff to monitor the labour and baby, and well-equipped to deal with any emergency. However, by the time that many mothers realize labour has started, organized the family, and contacted the hospital, the labour can be well under way.

The labour ward midwife who cares for you will inform the SCBU of your admission, giving them relevant details—your baby's gestation, your history, etc., enabling the SCBU to prepare an incubator and anticipate the equipment needed. The paediatrician is informed you are in labour and he will be contacted again when delivery is imminent. Ideally, a paediatrician is present at all preterm births ready to cope with any problems.

Monitoring in labour

During a preterm labour the ideal situation is to have a continuous record of the baby's heartrate so as to detect any deviation from normal. A small clip is attached to the baby's head, or on to the bottom of a breech baby. This is a small electrode which picks up impulses from the baby's heartbeat and these are transmitted along the connecting wires to be traced out on to paper as a graph of heartrate. The machine can be turned up so as the mother can hear the bleeps of the heartbeat, and a flashing light indicates each heartbeat.

Preparing for resuscitation

The labour ward always has resuscitation equipment available. When delivery is imminent a resuscitaire is brought into the delivery room. This is a portable piece of equipment which enables the doctor to have everything he could possibly require for immediate resuscitation of a newly born baby.

The resuscitaire houses oxygen and air cylinders with appropriate tubings, tiny masks and equipment to ventilate and assist breathing until the baby can be transferred to the SCBU. Suction is available to clear away mucus that may hinder breathing. Various drugs and drips are stored in a handy drawer. There is an overhead heater and lots of warm blankets to keep baby warm. A large stopwatch ticks away at the top of the resuscitaire, as time is vital in the first few minutes.

Forceps

Some doctors may deliver premature babies by forceps, the idea being that the forceps protect the baby's soft head from undue trauma. An episiotomy may also be done for the same reason. Other maternity units do not use forceps but believe that delivery by a skilled midwife or doctor is safer for the baby.

Current trends in childbirth are changing with more women taking an active role in the birth. When the baby is preterm much depends on the gestation of the baby, how she stands up to the stress of labour, and upon the condition of the mother.

Caesarean section

A Caesarean may be performed for a premature delivery. The actual operation to deliver a preterm baby by Caesarean section is identical to that for any birth. A paediatrician is in the theatre at all Caesarean births, prepared for any eventuality and, if possible at all, ensures that the mother sees her baby.

Retained placenta

When the birth is preterm it is more common for a placenta to refuse to come away from the wall of the uterus. This is called a retained placenta. Normal procedure is to give the mother an anaesthetic—general, epidural or a numbing injection. The doctor then manually removes the placenta.

Birth at home

The speedy arrival of many premature babies does mean that the birth can happen at home whilst waiting for the ambulance, midwife or doctor. This breech baby made an untimely entrance:

> The birth of our baby was a great shock in appalling conditions (in the hall of our flat). The flying squad only just arrived in time and my husband had to cope up to then.

The flying squad is a team consisting of an obstetrician, an anaesthetist, midwife and paediatrician who work within the hospital. When an obstetric emergency happens at home this team can be summoned and travels in a specially equipped ambulance to the home, ready to cope with any type of delivery or emergency situation. Mother and baby are brought into hospital—the baby travelling in a pre-heated travel incubator to keep her warm.

The baby

> As far as we're concerned, small is very beautiful!

A premature baby is now defined as a baby born before 37 weeks' gestation. A baby born at term, weighing less than 2500 g, is not preterm but is smaller than she should be, probably because she has not been nourished adequately while *in utero*. She is then referred to as 'light for dates'. However, just to complicate matters, preterm babies born before 37 weeks can also be light for dates! Weight is often expressed in metric; to help you convert to pounds and ounces there is a conversion chart at the end of the book (page 115).

Weight and maturity

Weight of the baby can bear little relevance to the maturity of the baby. It is maturity of baby that will determine how well she copes with the demands of her body and the outside environment. The earlier a baby is born the greater her problems can be expected to be, and the more immature her appearance will be.

Some babies can be a good weight and still have many problems because their bodies are too immature. For example, a baby born to a diabetic mother could weigh 9 lbs (4000g) and be of 34 weeks' gestation but have all the associated problems of any 34-week preterm baby.

What will my baby look like?

Your baby is *not* going to be a smaller version of a pink, chubby, full-term baby. She will *not* look like a typical baby in miniature. Parents are often unprepared for this.

Premature babies can look very 'foetal'. Obviously the more premature the baby the less like a full-term baby her appearance will be. Premature babies look skinny and wrinkled, and altogether frail, feeble, thin and helpless. Their skin colour will be very red, or a darkish red, or even very pale. The baby may have hair which is often shaved off in one or two patches, for medical reasons such as inserting a drip into the scalp vein; it may take a few months to regrow. Her eyes will usually be closed and may appear large in proportion to her face. Her arms are thin, and her legs may look oddly shaped as well as thin. Her bottom will appear odd and pointed. Her abdomen may seem too big, and her chest too small. Her navel seems to be oddly placed. The main reason for all these strange-looking features is that the premature baby was born before her fat stores could be laid down. This lack of fat can look off-putting, and is responsible for the frog-like bottom, thin bony face, and frail-looking arms. Limbs may be floppy, but tone and control will improve with maturity.

However, premature babies are usually perfectly formed. What you are seeing is not a *malformed* infant but a very *immature* one, with a body not yet finished getting ready for birth! She can cry, see, hear, and is sensitive to touch. Her inner organs are fully developed and do work—some inefficiently at first, but with help and a little time they soon become efficient.

It really is difficult to imagine how tiny a 2 lb (900 g) or 3 lb (1360 g) baby can be. To most people a newly born 8 lb (3630 g) baby seems very small. Look at your hand. Often the premature baby's finger is only the length of an adult finger nail!

Physical characteristics of a premature baby

At the time of birth, the baby was designed to be still floating in fluid inside the mother, and pressure from lying in one position gives her head a flattened appearance on one side.

The brain will develop more or less as it would within the womb, given good medical attention. On touching baby's head you will feel several soft areas where you would expect to feel a hard skull. These are normal in all babies and allow for growth of the brain. In premature babies the gaps between the head bones will feel wider compared with a full-term baby. These soft areas are called fontanelles.

The ears lack the cartilage which gives them their shape, so they will closely hug the sides of the head, and be easily pressed out of shape. Eyes are perfectly formed but may seem to bulge. Babies can open their eyes (except for extremely premature (24–25 weeks) babies, whose eyelids may still be fused). Eyebrows and lashes could be missing, but do not worry as this is common and they will grow within a few months.

All premature babies can make little noises and cry —however, it may sound very feeble and rather like a tiny kitten when compared to the loud cry of a larger baby.

> My baby daughter was born nine weeks early and weighed 3 lbs 4 oz (1470 g). She was unbelievably tiny. I was surprised that she looked so thin, like a nestling bird thrown out of her nest. Her head was the size of an orange. Her fingers were the same length as my husband's finger nails. Her legs were the thickness of his thumb. She looked as though you could hold her on an outstretched hand. She could have comfortably curled up in a box of tissues.

The abdomen will look large and the chest will look small.

Due to a lack of subcutaneous fat the ribs will show. If baby has breathing difficulties her chest may heave rather alarmingly, the ribs showing prominently. The baby could be making strange noises—grunting, wheezing, moaning noises associated with breathing problems. Once the condition is corrected the noises will stop, although her breathing may still cause obvious chest movements.

Baby's nipples are undeveloped—in many premature babies hardly visible at all. In time they will form and grow normally.

In boys the penis and scrotum are fully developed and, although small, will look normal. The testes may not have travelled down from inside the body into the scrotum. The doctor will check this, and reassure you that it is nothing to worry about in the early days as they probably will move down as baby matures.

In girls everything internally is perfectly formed, but externally the skin that forms the fleshy lips covering the entrance of the vagina may not have yet developed. This can make this area look abnormal, as the inner lips often protrude and can look swollen. In time the outer lips will grow and the area will look more normal.

In extremely premature babies the skin will look thin, shiny and almost transparent, and as the baby gets more mature the skin becomes tougher and more opaque. The blood vessels are near to the skin surface and clearly visible. A premature baby's skin is delicate and will bruise easily.

There could be a fine downy hair on baby's body, particularly on the face and back. This is called lanugo. It grows to protect the skin inside the uterus and is normally absorbed by the baby before birth. In preterm babies it may be present at birth, but it will go in time.

Because the baby should still be inside her mother floating in fluid, her body is not really designed to lie in one position and posture for long periods. Left to adopt their own position, most premature babies will take up a 'frog-like' position. They can move their limbs and in time will be able to alter position like a normal restless baby. Initially it is the nurses who will frequently change baby's position within the incubator and alter her posture. This prevents undue pressure on the baby's body.

All the systems within the body are perfectly formed but most work slowly and are sluggish in the early days. Much of this is due to weak muscles, the muscles working the intestines and urine system being unprepared for an early start.

Assessing gestational age

All low birth-weight babies are examined to assess their gestational age. This assessment is performed by an experienced paediatrician. The baby is undressed but kept warm within her incubator or under a suitable heater. By testing neurological responses, posture, tone, reflexes and body characteristics an accurate assessment can be made. There are several scoring systems which all assess gestational age, but the most widely used method is the Dubowitz system. The baby's gestational age is expressed in terms of weeks, full term being 40 weeks. At 28 weeks the foetus is viable, which means that, according to legal definition, it is capable of an independent existence and if born it must be registered. Despite this, tiny babies have been born at 23, 24, 25, 26 and 27 weeks' gestation and have survived, the vast majority of them growing into completely normal children. Given good medical care, 70 per cent of babies born at 27 or 28 weeks survive; 50 per cent of babies born at 26 weeks will survive; and babies have survived from 25, 24 and even 23 weeks. After 28 weeks the outlook is rosy—80 per cent of babies born at 29 weeks are surviving.[2] Babies born between 30 weeks and 37 weeks have virtually a 100 per cent chance of survival, with special medical care to prevent serious illness, and given that there are no major congenital defects.

Some facts and figures

In 1982 about 590,000[3] babies in this country were born alive. Of these 40,403 were babies with a low birth weight—that is, they each weighed 2500 g or less (about 5½ lbs). This amounts to almost 7 per cent of all babies. Of all these low birth-weight babies

69 per cent were in the heaviest group—2001–2500 g
31 per cent were 2000 g or less
3.8 per cent were 1000 g or less

It is interesting to compare the DHSS 1982 figures with those collected in 1966, less than 20 years ago. Here we show the percentage of babies surviving then and now, in each weight category:

Birth weight (grams)	*1966* (per cent)	*1982* (per cent)
1000 or less	15	40
1001—1500 g	51	83
1501—2000 g	86	95
2001—2250 g	95	98
2251—2500 g	97	99

In other words, 40 per cent of babies born weighing 2 lbs 3 oz (1000 g) or less are surviving. This figure rises to 83 per cent for babies weighing between 2 lbs 4 oz (1000) and 3 lbs 4 oz (1500 g). Ninety-five per cent of babies weighing between 3 lb 5 oz and 4 lb 6 oz (1501–2000 g) survive, and of babies born at weights greater than this only a very tiny percentage will *not* survive.

Overall, 94 per cent of all babies born weighing 5½ lbs (2500 g) or less are surviving, thanks to medical expertise and technology.

However, it will be seen that the more mature your baby is the better her chance of survival, and the easier her struggle against the difficulties caused by immature lungs and other organs.

The premature baby has a much better chance of survival nowadays than fifteen, ten, five or even two years ago, because of the very rapid growth of knowledge in neonatology, the study of newborn babies.

Will she be all right?

We have seen already that premature babies look quite different from full-term babies. Premature babies behave differently too. The question of behaviour and abilities of premature babies worries most parents. They are afraid that their baby might be brain-damaged, or retarded, or handicapped. This fear is quite normal and adds to the stress of a premature birth, but parents will be reassured to learn that the majority of even the tiniest surviving premature babies grow up to be perfectly normal, healthy, happy children.

Susan Goldberg and Barbara DiVitto have done much research into premature babies and their developmental abilities. They found from their studies that most premature babies—even tiny ones weighing between 1½ and 3¼ lbs (750 and 1500 g) grow up to be normal and healthy.[4] These normal healthy premature babies differ in many respects from full-term babies in their early development, but most of these differences disappear by the end of the first year.

The birth will have been traumatic for the baby, and she will have needed expert medical attention to ensure her survival. She will have been closely watched and nursed and will continue to be cared for in this way until her condition stabilizes. She is no longer a foetus, but a baby, born too soon admittedly but nevertheless a baby. Once her immediate struggle for survival is won, she will continue to grow and develop almost exactly as she would have done in the womb. Her brain will go through more or less the same developmental stages as it would have done *in utero*. Provided that she is receiving good intensive or special neonatal care, and loving, gentle attention from her parents, she will almost certainly grow to be the sort of child she would have been anyway, had her birth been at term. The task for the medical team is to give her as good a start as possible, by stabilizing her condition, and providing her with the environment she needs in which to survive and grow.

Good, constant communication with the baby's paediatrician is the key to minimizing worry. Talk as often as possible with the doctor. Show him that you are interested and informed and he will be open and honest with you.

Whether anticipated or not, the untimely arrival of a premature baby is still a great shock and only the beginning of a very anxious time ahead. It is a good idea to talk through all your experiences with someone close, and try mentally to prepare yourself for the next few weeks. Your premature baby, given good hospital care and parental love, has overall a 94 per cent chance of survival—although babies born before 29 weeks of pregnancy will obviously have a more difficult struggle. However early your baby, however frail and weak, she will benefit enormously from the medical technology available nowadays, and especially from her parents' care, contact and love.

TWO

After the Birth: How to Cope

First thoughts

> I remember registering the birth in the hospital—it seemed to be a challenge. She *did* exist, because she had been registered.

The time immediately following a premature birth is crucial. For the baby it often means a real struggle to survive. For the parents, the joy of childbirth is greatly reduced by worry and fear for their baby's life. For the mother, particularly, the first days are overloaded with stress, fear and anxiety. Her family is worried, friends and relatives are silent. The mother often feels guilty that she has failed to produce the kind of bouncing, healthy, robust baby shown in advertisements. Guilt that she has somehow caused her baby to suffer by his untimely arrival is a very common feeling. Medical staff, however, will reassure parents that a baby's prematurity is rarely related to anything the mother did, or didn't do, during pregnancy.

> When she was first born, I felt a sense of failure. Later, the failure turned to guilt, not only towards her, but also towards the rest of the family.

These feelings of guilt subside when the mother talks through her emotions with someone close, and she begins to realize that her tiny baby is not a reject but a little person in her own right, who happened to arrive too early, and who is receiving the best medical care possible to ensure her survival. Disbelief, shock and numbness are also very natural and common reactions to a premature birth.

It is important for parents to know that these emotional reactions are not only normal, but almost universal amongst mothers who have gone into premature labour and delivered a tiny, frail baby. Accepting these emotions and trying not to suppress them will make the struggle easier to bear. It is a good idea to be positive, but realistic. A good cry is therapeutic, as is talking through your worries with someone close. Accepting that your feelings of guilt, fear and anxiety are normal will help parents to face the situation with courage, rather than being submerged in despair.

> One's moods go up and down, terribly. I was encouraged by the staff to talk it all through, and to cry. You are mourning the child you *didn't* have, and are becoming accustomed to this pathetic bundle of problems. So I howled—and talked to anyone who would listen.

The fact that friends and relatives do not send their congratulations for fear of upsetting parents does little to encourage a positive approach to the newborn. Tiny, premature infants actually need their parents' love and attention even in the earliest days. It is far more beneficial to the baby, and to the parents, if a positive attitude is adopted. It is crucially important to accept and love even the tiniest of preterm babies, rather than letting natural fears and anxieties form a barrier between parent and child.

Back on the ward

> One had the feeling of being an embarrassment to the others. Visitors did not know what to say when they saw my empty bedside cot.

After the birth, the mother is usually separated from her premature baby, although more hospitals are now taking steps to keep mother and baby together by giving the mother a room attached to the special care unit. This is an ideal arrangement, as it encourages the mother to feel 'normal' and to feel comfortingly close to her newborn baby. It is government policy[5] now to recommend that mothers and premature babies are not separated, but kept as close as possible; however, most hospitals in the United Kingdom have not yet caught up with government recommendations for one reason or another. Sadly, it is still common for the mother to be taken back to the postnatal ward, without her precious baby, amongst all the other newly delivered mothers who have their babies with them.

The staff of a good maternity unit will consider the needs and feelings of mothers in this situation. Some are offered single rooms, and many nurses will ensure that the mother's need to talk and ask questions is catered for. It is a good idea to try to talk to the staff on the postnatal ward, and to ask questions about ward routine, doctors' rounds, mealtimes, etc., so that you can spend as much time as possible in the unit with baby, yet be in the right place at the right time for meals and medical examinations.

Of course, in some cases the mother is unable to visit her baby in the special care unit for one reason or another. This sometimes happens when certain medical problems arise. The mother may have been seriously ill with pre-eclampsia, or may not have made a normal recovery after a Caesarean section, particularly if it was an emergency operation. In these cases, during the short time that the mother is unable to be with her baby, she should be given plenty of support from the ward staff. Sick though the mother may be, she will still be concerned for her baby's health, and she will need constant news of the baby's progress. Photographs of the baby are often put at her bedside, and she will have visits from the paediatrician and SCBU staff who will talk with her about her baby. Some hospitals have a closed-circuit television service so that mothers can watch their baby continually on a portable TV screen by her bed. This is not a substitute for actually being with the baby, but it can be reassuring and can help bridge the awful gap of separation. One father we know took a video film of his daughter who was in an intensive care unit and replayed it to his wife who was in another hospital many miles away. This few minutes of film proved to be a source of reassurance and support to the mother until she could join her baby.

The first day or two after the birth is the time not only to rest and recover but also to begin to get to know the baby, even though she is in an incubator in the unit. Check with the ward staff that you can go to the SCBU to see your baby often, and begin to build up your relationship with her so that both you and the baby get the best possible start.

Seeing baby: the first time

> She opened her eyes and seemed to look right at me, she was so still and small and I felt these great waves of love and pity wash over me. I felt so helpless watching her struggle for life and the desire to scoop her up and hold her close to me was almost overwhelming. Instead, I put my arms over the incubator and cried my heart out, wanting somehow to pour my health and strength into her tiny frame.

As we have seen, a premature baby looks quite different from a full-term baby, her absence of body fat giving her a very thin, bony appearance, and this can be very upsetting for parents.

The baby seems overwhelmed by the technological trappings of the special care baby unit. It is normal to feel overawed, and even afraid, but the staff of a good SCBU will explain the functions of all the tubes and monitors, and will help parents to become accustomed to the machinery and to see beyond it to their baby.

Some mothers, through fear and lack of informed advice, are very reluctant to see their premature babies for the first time.

> I was moved back to the ward and put on a drip. How I prayed that the drip would stay, as I did not want to go and see my baby. I was afraid of what I would see.

This natural and common reluctance to see the premature baby for the first few times only stems from anxiety and fear. It helps to realize that the early preterm infant's struggle for survival is actually eased by parental cuddling, stroking, and gentle caressing. Once parents understand that a premature baby is as much in need of their love and attention as a full-term infant, they can manage to overcome their anxieties and make a positive move to build up a loving relationship with their baby.

If it is at all possible, parents can benefit enormously from holding and cuddling their babies at the earliest opportunity. The staff will meet the mother and father and will explain the medical equipment in the unit. Parents should take this opportunity to ask questions about their baby, to try to gain as much information as possible about the unit, and to ask about the feasibility of cuddling their baby, even briefly.

> I held his one free hand and when I felt a tiny grip on my fingers I just prayed he would get stronger.

Some mothers worry that they do not feel a surge of love for their premature baby. Anxiety and stress can combine to diminish the natural rush of emotion experienced by so many mothers. It is hardly surprising, given the circumstances, that anxious, overwrought parents seeing their premature babies for the first time feel rather less than ecstatic.

Konrad Lorenz[6] demonstrated that babies have tremendous powers to initiate response in adults, just by their physical appearance. He showed that the newborn and very young babies of animals, including puppies and kittens—and human babies—all have in common a set of physical features which combine to evoke a favourable response from us. They possess a large head, and a cute cluster of features which we find appealing—and parents, looking down at their long-awaited chubby newborn babies, respond positively with smiles and pleasure. But the premature infant, especially one born very early, does not possess the cute, appealing features characteristic of the full-term baby. She can look thin and scrawny, out of proportion, and bony. It is no wonder then that some mothers are unable to fall instantly in love with their premature babies, when they describe them as: 'A chicken without its feathers' or 'Just a bag of bones'. Even the photographs taken by SCBU staff of the baby in his incubator and given to the mother to keep by her bedside, often give little indication of reality.

These reactions are normal and understandable. But it is reassuring to know that as the baby grows fitter and more mature, she puts weight on steadily and she begins to look more like a full-term infant, with chubby cheeks, plump arms, legs and bottom.

Encouraged by SCBU staff, parents can touch and stroke their baby, hold and cuddle her, and gradually begin to take over some of the caretaking duties, like changing and feeding. This actual physical contact is the foundation of a solid, loving relationship.

> Seeing him in the incubator soon after the birth, I felt he wasn't mine and that I hadn't just given birth to him . . . 24 hours later when I held him and changed him I felt a great surge of love for this poor bruised and bloody-headed little thing.

Building a relationship

> Holding, cuddling, talking to a newborn baby all the time, no matter how ill or small he is, is just as important as all the fancy machinery. It gives him strength to fight.

The special care baby unit is a specially equipped and heated ward for sick newborn and premature babies. It contains modern technological gadgets and monitors which help the highly trained staff continually to assess and tend their tiny patients. The specially trained doctors and nurses who work on the SCBU would certainly be amongst the first to assure parents of preterm babies that however modern the technology, however efficient the medical service, it is the *parents* who are central to the care of the sick newborn (see also Chapter 3). Indeed, premature babies in an under-equipped hospital in Bogotá are carried snugly inside the mother's clothing, next to her breast.

The old idea of the baby being separated from her family in order to prevent the risk of infection is now no longer held to be valid. The more the mother can do for her own baby, the better. If parents can take over much of the daily care of their premature baby, even while she is still in the incubator, they can reduce the risk of cross-infection, and the baby can acquire maternal bacterial flora which may prevent colonization by pathogenic hospital strains.[7]

> Special care cannot be just clinical as if the baby were a faulty machine; it has to be personal and to care for the whole family,

> because the family will be responsible for the baby during the next few vulnerable years.[8]

It is a prime task for the SCBU team to encourage parents to visit, to participate, and to join in with the everyday routine, although some units are very busy and undermanned. It is also a good idea for parents to show the staff that they are keen to participate in the care of their infant.

It is an enormous help to parents to have written information about the special care baby unit, in the form of a specially written leaflet explaining the machinery, and the routine. Although a recent survey[9] showed that 69 per cent of SCBUs have written information available, only 5 per cent of our sample were actually given leaflets or booklets. Most doctors and nurses are happy to explain the monitors, tubes and wires personally to the parents, but many SCBU staff simply forget that the technology is unfamiliar to strangers and omit to explain it unless specifically asked. Some of the parents in our sample stressed that asking questions is absolutely necessary. We strongly suggest that you ask questions over and over again until you are satisfied.

Much has been said during recent years about bonding, and how a lack of bonding between mother and baby at birth is supposed to have a detrimental subsequent effect on their relationship. It is true that many mothers experience a sort of ecstatic rush of emotion when they see their newborn baby—and it is also true that many do not, whether the baby is premature or full-term. Mothers of premature babies are far less likely to feel unalloyed joy, because of the stress, anxiety, and fear of their baby's death. However, we have found that whether the ecstasy is there or not a mother-baby attachment can be as strong and binding as ever with premature babies.

> To be honest there was no surge of motherly love, in fact I had to convince myself that this tiny baby in the incubator was mine and had come from me . . . As she grew stronger I suppose my feelings did too.

It is through cuddling and caring that mother–baby

attachment is likely to strengthen, even given the shaky start of a sudden premature birth. Withdrawing from the baby will never help. If the baby lives, she will need her mother's love right from the first minute. If she dies, despite all the medical help given, the mother will find it easier to mourn a child she knew and loved, rather than an unseen stranger. Fear that your baby will die is natural, but it is important to face the fear squarely, and try to accept it, rather than push it to the back of your mind. Having accepted that you are afraid of your baby's death, you may then feel able to visit her, hold her, cuddle her, talk to her, and build up a relationship based on love rather than fear.

There is no doubt whatsoever that early contact with a premature baby does help the mother form an attachment, and that the more time parents spend with their baby in the SCBU the more solid their relationship. There are many things parents can do at the baby's side, even if she is in an incubator, or even on ventilation.

Most SCBU staff nowadays will encourage parents to open the incubator portholes and stroke their baby, gently and caressingly—stroke her soft body, and touch her fingers and toes. The baby may move her arms and legs in response to your soft touch, and she may turn her head if you stroke her cheek. It has been found that the clinical handling by staff for tests or treatment distresses the sick premature baby, and that those vital oxygen levels fall on each occasion. Researchers, however, have concluded that gentle fondling and quiet, soft caressing strokes may reduce the number of 'forgetting to breathe', or apnoea, attacks in a premature baby, may help weight gain, and may help increase transcutaneous oxygen values.[10]

> The hardest times were finding him crying so pitifully inside his oxygen hood. Touching and stroking seemed to help us both.

It is a good idea to check with the nurse that you can open the incubator porthole to stroke your baby—you will probably find the staff encouraging and helpful in this respect. A baby is never too ill that you can't even hold her hand.

There is little doubt that talking to your baby is beneficial for all concerned. The baby will learn to identify her parents' voices, and talking is, after all, a basic social factor essential in forming relationships. Talk calmly to your baby, bring her a musical mobile or toy, and she will learn to respond. The only exception to this is when you are establishing feeding. She will feed better if you are quiet and calm. Save the talking for another time.

Holding and cuddling

The staff will often ask if you want to hold your baby—they will never jeopardize baby's health, but they recognize that parental holding and cuddling is so important for both baby and parents.

> We finally got to hold him after just two days. What with all the monitors for heartbeat, blood gases, respiration, ventilators and drips—we did a careful but joyous juggling act.

When you are holding your baby, loosen her blankets a little so that she is not wrapped so tightly. Tickle her toes, and talk to her. Gradually she will wake up, and when her eyes are open, bring your face close to within 9 inches (22 cm) of her face. She may look at you and follow you with her eyes.

In our sample many mothers brought a small, brightly coloured toy to hang near their baby, and one mother brought photographs of the baby's older siblings and stuck them on the incubator, on strict instructions from her two small sons who insisted that their tiny sister should recognize them when she came home! Another mother brought photographs of the baby's new nursery bedroom at home, newly decorated and prepared, for her baby to look at in the incubator. Being positive and open is good for everyone.

Caring for your baby

Good neonatal units encourage mothers, and fathers, to participate in the daily care of their baby. Parents are taught by staff to change baby's nappy, clean her face and hands, take her temperature, change her resting position, and sometimes to feed their baby themselves via the nasogastric tube. It is generally felt by researchers in this field that a baby benefits tremendously from individualized care, rather than being cared for routinely by a number of different nurses. This is easily accomplished if the mother is rooming-in with her baby on the unit. If it is at all possible for the mother to stay in the unit, as is quite often the case when the baby is a first baby, then she should make use of the residential facilities available. Some units have special bedrooms for use by mothers. And many of these bedrooms are underused—parents simply do not realize that they are for mothers if they wish to stay. Ask about rooming-in arrangements if you can—this will enable you to participate in the daily care of your premature baby. Staying close to your baby, and being as actively involved as possible in her daily care, will be of great benefit to all concerned and can only serve to give the baby—and mother—the best possible start.

Fathers

When a baby is born too soon, for whatever reason, it is often the father who is most involved at the very beginning. Sometimes the father is present at the birth, even if it is a Caesarean section. Sometimes though, if the birth is sudden and quick, or if the Caesarean is an emergency, he cannot reach his wife in time to see his baby being born. This is often a disappointment to both parents. However, in many ways, the father then becomes much more involved with his premature baby than if the baby was born at term. The mother may need time to recover from her Caesarean, or from her pre-eclampsia, and in these cases the father can get to know the special care unit before the mother. In this respect he can do much to prepare the mother for her first visit to the unit, and of course he can make the first contact with the baby and begin to build up the family bond.

> My husband saw him first and—instant love! They are still closely bonded.

Many special care baby units encourage fathers right

from the start to participate in the baby's care—some are beginning to provide beds for them. The whole emphasis nowadays, thankfully, is on parental involvement and establishing a family bond. Gone are the days when, as one of our mothers remembered, fathers who attempted to visit their premature babies in the unit were frogmarched back down the corridor by bustling nurses with the firm rebuff 'Fathers are *not* allowed in the Nursery. They might be *dirty*!'

These early days are full of strain and worry for both parents. It is important to talk out your feelings with each other, so that you can face the turbulent weeks together, strongly, rather than harbouring resentment and hiding your sorrow. The whole experience of having a premature baby can put a strain on family life.

We strongly advise that both parents share their feelings with each other, and try to help each other to stay positive and strong. Use the strength of your relationship as ballast during these first weeks, and you will come through the experience maybe a little wiser and, best of all, together.

Baby's progress

Once your baby's condition has been assessed, treatment begins immediately to help her survive and grow. She will gain strength day by day until she is ready to be discharged. She may be in special care for a week or so, or for several weeks or even months, depending on her condition. It is important to remember that the hospital wants to see your baby fit and healthy and feeling well before she goes home, but to some parents the wait is almost unbearable, and their baby's progress is uncomfortably erratic.

This is a very difficult time for parents. Our advice is to try hard to see things in perspective. The medical staff are as anxious as you to see your baby growing healthy and ready to go home. Try to take each day as it comes, and rejoice when your baby makes a little progress.

While your baby is in the SCBU she is receiving excellent medical care. Use this time to get to know the routine, and the staff, and try to talk as much as possible with the nurses. Show that you are interested in their work, and build up a good relationship with them. This will help you to feel confident and welcomed, and it will help the staff—who after all, work in an extremely stressful environment—to look forward to your visits, knowing that you care. A pleasant, caring atmosphere is ideal for staff, parents—and your baby.

Going home—without your baby

Some time after the birth, the mother is judged well enough by the obstetrician to be discharged. She can then join her baby, if possible, on the SCBU, making use of the residential facilities available. If she is unable to do this, she will go home, leaving her baby in special care. This is still the commonest situation—and it can be a very distressing one. For many mothers it means the dilemma of wanting to be in two places at once, particularly if there are older children in the family.

> I felt very torn—I wanted to be at the hospital all the time but I also needed to be at home with my two other children, aged four and two, as they needed extra comfort at this time.

Obviously, if there are other children to be cared for while the baby is still in special care, then the parents must work out the best way they can to cope with their own particular situation. Again, try to put things in perspective. Things like housework, shopping and cooking can be done by any willing helpers. Friends and family will want to help all they can, and this is an ideal time to make use of any offers. Try to use your own time to be with your children and the baby. With older children, be loving and extra affectionate, for they too will be feeling the strain. Depending on their age and maturity, they can participate in the family concern for the new, frail baby. Talk about the baby, in her incubator, explain in simple terms about the special care unit. Let them draw pictures, and encourage conversation. Take them to see their tiny new sister or brother—and, in general, involve them. They will feel less lonely and confused, and they will be much happier. Of course, if you feel unable to talk to your children in this way or if they are too young then try at least to be happy and positive with them. If you are visiting the unit every day, make sure that your children are cared for by someone close in your absence. They will need extra love and attention from everyone.

There is no doubt that leaving your baby in special care once you have been discharged is distressing. Even the most motivated and caring of parents begin to feel the exhaustion and strain of constant worry, and countless visits to the unit. The feelings of panic only stem from love and concern for the baby. Your anxieties can be eased by having confidence in the SCBU team, by talking to them, asking questions, and by being there as much as possible. Sometimes the visits seem a total waste of time; travelling up to 60 miles (100 kilometres) to sit and watch a tiny baby fighting for her life does seem futile. If you have to stay at home and the hospital is a great distance away, you should talk over the situation with your partner, and the SCBU staff. Obviously it is best for the baby—and for you—that you stay near her as much as possible, but if the cost in terms of stress is too great, then you have to re-examine your plans. Ask about residential facilities on the SCBU or in the hospital itself. Talk to the paediatrician, explain your problems, and try to work out a solution which is good for all of you.

Getting help

At this difficult time, parents need a lot of help and support. Friends and relatives who offer help should never be turned away. Use their kindness to alleviate your daily work routine and spend time with your children and partner. There are other sources of help too—all addresses are at the end of the book, page 111.

National Childbirth Trust (NCT)
The NCT has been of enormous help to many parents of special care babies. Local branches can often put you in touch with someone who has faced the same problems, and

who will be glad to talk over the situation with you. They can also loan you an electric or manual breast pump, for a small fee, and they have breastfeeding counsellors who are trained to be knowledgeable about the whole business of expressing milk. They publish leaflets which may help, and can be a tremendous moral support.

National Association for the Welfare of Children in Hospital (NAWCH)
This Association is very interested in special care babies and will be keen to help if you contact them. They too can offer moral support, and can give you information about SCBUs and premature babies.

Parent support groups
There is now a national support group called 'Nippers' for families with babies in special care, but many hospitals run their own parent support groups attached to their own SCBUs. Ask if your SCBU has one, and contact them for extra support and information.

Department of Health and Social Security
The DHSS may be able to help you with travel costs to visit your baby in hospital. The costs mount up if you are visiting your baby daily for, say, two months. One mother calculated that she spent £90 on petrol. If you do not have a car, your fares may be expensive. Contact your local DHSS and see if you qualify for help. If they cannot give you financial assistance we suggest that you try the local branch of NAWCH, or ask to talk to the hospital social worker. She may know where you can get help.

Department of Employment
When a baby is born prematurely, especially if born say at 26 weeks, a working mother will need extra time away from her job. You have the right to stay away from work until your baby is 29 weeks old. In normal cases, the baby would then be about seven months old, but a 26-week premature baby will be the equivalent of around four months. You can, in special circumstances, extend your maternity leave, but

only by a maximum of four weeks. To do this, contact the Department of Employment in your area. The booklet *Employment Rights for the Expectant Mother*, published by the Department of Employment, gives full details of how to extend your maternity leave.

Keeping your outlook positive

While your baby is in special care, try to use the time wisely and positively. You will probably be expressing milk and spending as much time as you can in the SCBU but you can also use this time to prepare for your baby's homecoming, to catch up on sleep, and to organize yourself generally. One mother in our sample used this time to contact her local clinic, to ask about attending some parentcraft classes. One mother kept a diary of her baby's progress, and each day's joys and frustrations. This is a good idea—it can be a way of expressing your emotions instead of bottling them up, and it gives you a concrete record of the weeks in SCBU. Many mothers in our sample felt themselves lucky to have some time to regain their strength and get organized, before baby's discharge. We think this is important, as any new baby creates a tremendous amount of work, and often premature babies can be very unsettled in their first few months at home. This is quite normal, but hard work nevertheless.

> I can look back and see some advantages in Katy's prematurity. I got 6 weeks of sleeping through the night without interruption, so I had recovered physically from the birth by the time she came home.

When your baby is on the road to recovery and is growing more mature and bigger each day, your hopes begin to rise. You can see the light at the end of the tunnel. You are beginning to look back and remember the birth, the shock, and the fear, and you are able to see them more in perspective. No-one can deny that having, say, a 26-week preterm baby is the most emotionally draining experience you are likely to have in your lifetime. But you *do* recover, and you emerge from the experience a little sadder, a little wiser, and with a more mature outlook on life. This mother was able to remember her SCBU experiences objectively, and her advice is invaluable.

> My general advice is, ask questions, however obvious they may seem. The more interest you show, the better the relationship with the SCBU staff, and so the more they will tell you. Look on yourself as part of the caring team—the most important part. Show lots of interest and enthusiasm, and enjoy all the experiences, as they'll help you learn, and grow.

THREE

After the Birth: The Special Care Baby Unit

> I can never find the words to express my gratitude and appreciation to all the staff, the doctors' dedication is wonderful —in a strange way I will be sad to leave all the kind people as I now regard them as friends. I could not have wished my baby to be anywhere else, I think he received love, kindness and medical attention that would be hard to beat. I thank the staff of the SCBU for my son's life.

Special care baby units (SCBU) are special wards in maternity hospitals for babies who need extra care after birth. The unit is supervised by a paediatrician—a doctor who has special training in the care of babies and children. The nurses are experienced and skilled in the nursing of small and ill babies.

Many babies need extra care after birth—10 per cent of *all* babies will spend time on a SCBU, so as well as premature babies you may see other babies with different problems. Parents are encouraged to spend as much time as possible on the unit with their baby and family-centred care is now advocated in many units.

SCBUs are becoming welcoming places—'Your Baby Needs You—and so do we!' is a notice displayed in one SCBU. The units may be brightly decorated, with murals and friezes, and the staff are welcoming and friendly. Our survey revealed that most parents had nothing but praise for the high quality of care their babies had received.

Mobiles, bright posters, gaily painted walls all help to detract from the 'intensive' atmosphere created by all the necessary equipment. Notice-boards full of information, before and after photographs of babies from the unit, plants, comfortable waiting and rest rooms all do help to create a less formal and more welcoming atmosphere, at a time when parents are under maximum stress.

Any mother who has recently given birth to her much longed-for baby, naturally wants to be with or near to the baby. If the facility is available, staying near to your baby is the ideal situation.

Family-centred care

Many SCBUs now actively encourage the parents to be involved in the care of their baby's everyday needs, showing them what they can do, where things are kept and how to hold, touch and care for their baby.

Involving parents in care can range from changing a nappy to tube feeding. The nurses will show you, more than once if necessary, how to cope with changing nappies around monitoring tubes, washing a tiny little face and generally how to care for a baby in an incubator. In the early days it may only be possible to touch your baby, but as she gets stronger there should be no limitation in involving parents in care.

It may seem a frightening prospect for the mother at the start of baby's stay in SCBU to be involved in caring for her baby, who may seem a tiny scrap of body surrounded by numerous wires, tubes and machinery. As she loses the tubes, grows and moves from incubator to a cot and then home to her family, the confidence and skills you will have learnt on the SCBU will be helpful in the early days at home.

> We were always allowed to do everything for her in hospital, including tube feeding and administering drugs and so when we came to bring her home we felt totally confident.

The baby

In the initial period following admission to the baby unit, or when the baby is ill, it is advantageous to nurse the baby naked. Within the incubator or under a radiant heater she can be kept warm and comfortable. The staff can observe and care for her with minimal disturbance. Seeing your baby naked and sprawled out within an incubator can be very upsetting. It is your natural instinct to protect and provide security.

The baby may lie on a small sheepskin blanket; these are commonly used in SCBUs. Usually made of lambswool or a synthetic fibre, they provide a soft, warm and comfortable bedding for baby to lie on. Research[11] shows that babies nursed on sheepskin-type blankets rest and sleep easier, save energy and oxygen by reduced movement and consequently gain weight faster than babies nursed on cotton sheets.

As the baby's condition improves she will be dressed in some sort of clothing. Thankfully, most units have abandoned the standard ill-fitting hospital nightclothes and vests, and now can provide a wide range of clothes specially made for tiny babies. The baby will wear a dress, nightie, or baby suit depending on what the unit has available and she may even wear a hat and bootees. A well-fitting woolly hat helps in keeping the baby warm as much body heat is lost from the head.

Telephoning the unit

> . . . we could telephone at any time. I always phoned before I went to bed. All staff were concerned for all the family from consultant to nurse and I never felt in the way.

When you are at home without your baby it is only natural to worry and become concerned for baby. It is all too easy to let these feelings get out of proportion—so do telephone the unit and be reassured. Any time, day or night, the staff will always be only too glad to talk with you about your baby's condition. However, it is advisable for only the parents to telephone the unit so try to encourage other family members to ring you at an appropriate time at home.

SCBU routines

Your baby will start her stay in SCBU being nursed in an incubator—then she will be moved perhaps to a heated cot and afterwards to an ordinary cot. Each move will probably be accompanied by a move into a less intensive nursery room.

The day-to-day nursing care of your baby will depend on

how ill she is, how much staff instigate family-centred care and the policies within the unit.

Washing or bathing the baby takes place daily, as does renewal of equipment where necessary. Eye cleaning, mouth care and changing nappies happen many times within a day, and hopefully parents are encouraged to do these things whenever possible.

Babies are fed frequently initially—small amounts every hour at first, progressing to two-hourly and then three-hourly feeds. Once the baby is much stronger breast or bottle feeding can be established on demand. The sister-in-charge assesses all the baby's feed daily, the amount depending on weight gain, type of milk and how well or badly baby is feeding.

The doctors have a daily visit to all the babies—'a doctors' round'. All the doctors on the unit and some of the nurses and other professional staff are involved. Each baby is assessed and alterations made to nursing or medical care, tests ordered or results discussed and the baby's records kept up to date. This is when most decisions are made.

The staff often have meetings to discuss the babies, methods of care and how to improve individual babies' well-being.

Weighing

The babies are all weighed frequently. In some units this can be daily, in others three to four times a week.

Weight is used to calculate amount of feeds, fluid balance, amounts of medicines and, of course, show progress by weight gain. Initially, weight loss is expected. The more ill the baby the longer she will be in regaining her birth weight. When baby develops an illness, weight gain is often temporarily halted.

Try not to put too much emphasis on weight gain in the early days—your baby's fitness and general health is of first importance.

Some units stipulate that a certain weight goal must be reached before the baby can be discharged. Usually this is 4½ lbs (2040 g) or 5 lbs (2270 g).

Blood tests

Premature babies will have many blood tests. The blood is taken by several methods, the three most common being:

1 *Heelprick*—a small amount of blood is taken from the heel of the baby. Alternate heels are used each time and the subsequent 'scarring' will fade in time.

2 *From a vein*—where more blood is required than 1 ml (millilitre), a small needle is inserted into a vein, common sites being the head, back of the hand, and arm.

3 *From an artery*—an artery is a blood vessel that has fresh oxygen in it, and when blood is needed to assess the blood gases it is taken by a small needle from an artery in the wrist or top of the leg. Blood can also be taken from an artery in the umbilical cord.

Intravenous infusion (drips)

Ill premature babies may require a drip. It may be to give fluid, to give drugs or to feed the baby. The drip is set up by a doctor who prescribes the fluid your baby is to receive. A drip can be positioned anywhere on baby's body where a vein is close to the skin surface. Places commonly used on babies are veins in the head, arms and feet. The veins on the head are the largest in the body and easiest to use. This position will involve shaving off a small area of hair—but it will grow again in a few months.

Drips can look very uncomfortable but if correctly positioned should not upset the baby too much. Often the tapes, cottonwool padding, splints, etc. used to keep the drips in position and comfortable make the drip look very large compared to the baby. The fine plastic tube in the vein is easily disturbed and removed. SCBU staff get quite ingenious at devising various methods of securing the drips in position.

Suction tubes

It is necessary to have suction facilities near each intensive care cot and in each nursery room. Modern hospitals have a suction unit attached to a wall next to the oxygen outlet, older hospitals will use a suction machine.

A disposable sterile suction tube is attached to the main length of tube originating from the source of suction. This can be gently used to remove mucus, excess water, regurgitated milk, etc. from the baby's mouth and tiny air passages, to let her breathe normally.

Charts and records

The nurses keep detailed charts to show baby's progress, usually on a clipboard near to the incubator or cot. There are many different charts, which vary in format and content. The nurses can chart anything from feeding, weight gain, drip rates, heart beat, apnoea attacks, jaundice, etc.—the list is endless. If you are interested in your baby's charts the nurses will usually not mind explaining them to you.

SCBU equipment

> Initially the machinery etc. was frightening but the staff reassured us what the normal readings were and in the end the sight of drips, alarms etc. became a way of life.

SCBUs and neonatal intensive care units (NICUs) are full of expensive, technological and perhaps intimidating-looking equipment. It is quite normal to feel anxious at the sight of all the equipment around your baby. Staff should explain what it all is for, and if you can understand this it will help to allay a lot of fear.

The nurses will show how and where to touch your baby amidst her mass of tubes and wires. They understand how difficult this must be for you the first time and help you manoeuvre your hand to make physical contact with your baby. It is important to establish contact and only in extremely rare situations will this not be permitted. Given time, you will soon start to familiarize yourself with the sight of the equipment, leads, probes and wires, and learn to cope quite easily handling your baby without disturbing the equipment.

The incubator

Incubators hold no magical properties, and should not place any 'barriers' between parents and their babies.

In the incubator the baby can be seen and watched clearly without disturbance. Warmed, humidified air, and oxygen if required, can be given. The baby is kept warm at an ideal temperature controlled by the baby's own body temperature. Intensive care can be given to the baby or she can be nursed without any monitors or attachments in an ideal environment.

What is an incubator?

The base is a metal cupboard on wheels which allows access from both sides. The baby's personal linen, nappies, cottonwool, washing bowls, etc. are kept in this cupboard. On top of the cupboard is a simple fan and heating system and a control panel. Above the control panel is the incubator top—a large, perspex box. It has several round opening doors large enough to put your hand and arm through. Known as portholes, these allow access to baby without losing too much heat and oxygen. Each long side of the top is hinged and lets down to allow clear access to the baby, and the ends also drop down. There are many small grooves and holes around the portholes and doors to allow tubes, monitor wires, etc. inside the incubator.

The baby lies inside on a small table, which can be raised at either end if necessary or be left flat, on a soft mattress, a sheet or a sheepskin blanket.

Babies can stay in incubators for days or many weeks depending on their size, maturity and state of health.

Travel incubators are used for transporting very ill babies from one hospital to another. They are smaller than the incubator in the SCBU, and can be lifted into the ambulance and secured for travelling to the other hospital. While in transit babies can be given oxygen, ventilated and monitored.

Radiant heaters

Babies in neonatal intensive care units who are very ill can be nursed in the open but under a large radiant heater. Monitoring equipment, ventilator, etc. will surround them. Once the condition improves, the baby can be moved into an incubator.

Heated cot

When she can maintain her own body temperature and is well enough, the baby will be moved from her incubator into a cot and usually a slightly cooler nursery room. The cot may be heated by a small strip radiant heater over the top of the cot. It may be a specially designed heated cot or a standard perspex cot with metal frame and a heater unit placed over the top. Modern cots have a cupboard under them in which to keep baby's personal linen, nappies and her bath.

The baby will now be dressed, but may still have some equipment with her, such as an apnoea alarm (to monitor the baby's breathing). She will be snugly wrapped in blankets and perhaps an attractive overquilt.

Heat shields

If baby is cold a heat shield can be put temporarily over the top of the cot. A heat shield is a thick perspex sheet that fits exactly on to the cot—rather like a lid. It has several holes for ventilation. If baby remains cold it may be necessary to move her back into an incubator.

Heat shields are commonly used in incubators—either a head box heat shield which fits over baby's head and keeps the warmed oxygenated air in, or a rounded heat shield placed over the baby's body. Rounded shields are used on very ill babies nursed under radiant heaters.

Monitors

Ideally, it is important to be able to check the baby's progress continually without disturbing the baby. Premature babies may be monitored for many weeks, but this may not mean they are seriously ill.

Most monitoring is done by attaching small sticky-backed discs to the baby's skin. These discs are attached to wires which go to the individual pieces of monitoring equipment. The discs (or probes) pick up electrical impulses, heat, breathing movements, etc., depending on their function—and it is related and transmitted on the relevant monitor. The discs do not hurt or harm the baby, and can sometimes come unstuck causing an alarm to ring and alert the nurses.

Infection in SCBUs

Fear of infection in a SCBU is the concern of the staff. Infections can make babies seriously ill and an outbreak of infection can close a unit down temporarily. Premature babies and ill babies are at risk and vulnerable to many germs. An SCBU, being hot and humid, is an ideal breeding ground for bacteria. High rates of infection are found in SCBUs when compared with other hospital wards. Awareness of the way infections are caused leads the staff to be extra careful in preventing them.

Babies with infections are given antibiotics and some units routinely give prophylactic (preventive) antibiotics to all babies to prevent infection.

How you can help prevent infection

Handwashing is important. You will be encouraged to wash your hands when you enter the nursery room and before handling baby. The sinks have no plugs, as these are germ traps. Antiseptic solution commonly replaces soap. Taps are elbow taps. Towels are paper and disposable. Encourage your visitors and children to wash their hands before touching the baby.

Gown and mask wearing is a controversial issue. Gowns do not reduce infection rates and many units do not expect parents to wear them. Plastic aprons (disposable) are more generally acceptable to protect your clothes when caring for baby.

Personal items belonging to your baby, such as bedding linen, nappies, clothes, bath, bowl, etc. are all kept in the incubator base or base of her cot. Try to keep them there and not spread around the room. If anything falls on to the floor ask the nurse for a clean replacement.

Try to make it your responsibility to see that people planning to visit you and your baby are in good health, and not suffering from colds or coughs, or other illnesses.

The staff

A well-run, happy and efficient SCBU depends largely upon the smooth interaction of many people. Doctors and nurses work together, liaising with a large back-up team ranging from X-ray staff to the cleaners.

Different hospitals have different uniforms for nurses, with various distinguishing features. Staff turnover may be high, but faces will soon start to become familiar.

Asking questions

We cannot stress enough the importance of asking—again and again. When you feel you can understand what is happening to your baby coping becomes easier, even though you may feel you get negative answers to your queries at first. 'How long will my baby be in hospital?' and 'Will she be all right?' are the two hardest questions to answer. Generally, the more ill your baby or the more prematurely she was born, the longer her length of stay on SCBU will be. Try to take each hour at a time. The staff should understand the stresses and strains put upon parents.

Being with your baby

Recognizing the importance of maximum parental contact, 93 per cent[12] of SCBUs allow unlimited, unrestricted parental access over 24 hours. Access by other members of the family—brothers and sisters, grandparents, close family members—varies between units. Thankfully, the trend is to encourage family visiting. Ask what the arrangements are, especially for grandparents and siblings.

Ideally, the mother should be able to stay near to her baby in the SCBU or hospital, but as this is not always possible or practical, every encouragement must be made for parents to visit baby, either together or separately.

The SCBU staff are there to help you all they can; they do understand when visiting is difficult. Talk to them about problems and often help can be given or the best arrangements made for you to be with your baby.

Parents' sitting-rooms are an advantage on a SCBU. They can often be decorated, furnished and equipped through voluntary organizations or charities. They can include notice and photo boards, a toy cupboard for children, a small library shelf for parents and children.

> There was a room for mums in the SCBU where we could make drinks, courtesy of NAWCH, and chat between feeds. At times it was exhausting listening to everyone's problems though we knew we all supported each other, shared the good news and the bad.

When not to come to the SCBU

The only time you will be asked not to visit is when you are ill. The baby is very vulnerable to infection. An adult cold may be irritating, but to a preterm baby it could be a very serious illness. If you have a cough, cold, spots or diarrhoea, or any other illness, play safe and ring the unit before you visit and consult the sister for advice.

FOUR

Medical Problems

All preterm babies will require some medical care—whether it is minimal or intensive depends on the baby's prematurity and condition. Generally, the more preterm the baby was born, the more intensive will be the care required. Intensive care units specifically for babies, with all the experienced medical and back-up staff, equipment and staff skilled in using it, providing 24-hour care for seriously ill babies, are not common. They are usually only found in the larger city hospitals, making it necessary for the majority of babies requiring intensive care to be transferred from SCBU to a neonatal intensive care unit (NICU) in another hospital, often many miles away. Babies return to the SCBU once intensive care is no longer necessary.

Heat control—why do premature babies get cold?

Premature babies lack body fat—not only the subcutaneous fat under the skin that helps to keep us warm, but also brown fat. Brown fat is a special fat in our bodies found at the base of the neck, between the shoulder blades and around the kidneys. In the premature baby it is only present in small amounts compared to the amounts found in a full-term baby. Brown fat can supply energy quickly to the body to be used for heat production, so the premature baby is at a disadvantage. In fact, the part of the brain which controls the baby's response to body temperature is not mature enough to function properly. The task of the medical team is to keep the baby's temperature stable, and to prevent chilling or overheating.

After birth, the baby is dried quickly, wrapped in warm towels and, if condition allows, a quick cuddle with mother and father. The baby is taken to the SCBU to be settled into a warm environment. Many units use large shaped sheets of a specialized foil—called a 'space blanket' or 'silver swaddler'—which acts as an insulator during transfer of the baby.

Body and environmental temperatures are monitored continually until the ideal is reached. The extremely premature or ill baby—both will have great difficulty in keeping warm—may be nursed under a large radiant heater. To keep heat and humidified air in, a rounded perspex heat shield or a special plastic sheet is placed over the baby. The humidified air stops baby's body surface from drying out.

Breathing difficulties—why do premature babies find it difficult to breathe?

Ten per cent of premature babies will experience breathing difficulties, the highest incidence occurring in those weighing 900 to 1500 g. Breathing difficulties are anticipated in premature babies because of the lungs' immaturity and difficulty in adapting to life outside the mother.

Respiratory distress syndrome (RDS)

Respiratory distress syndrome occurs shortly after birth or up to four hours later. The baby cannot expand the lungs properly and so fails to receive adequate oxygen which is needed for normal body functions. Carbon dioxide is the body's waste gas and is usually exchanged in the lungs for fresh oxygen—and then breathed out. When it is not removed it begins to accumulate in the baby's body. She starts to 'fight' to obtain fresh oxygen and quickly becomes ill. The severity of the respiratory distress will vary depending on how much surfactant is present in the baby's lungs. The baby looks very ill, breathing is rapid and accompanied by a grunting, whining or rasping noise. The nostrils flare and the baby can be a blue-grey colour. Breathing is difficult so that the baby uses different muscles to help the lungs work, causing her chest to heave, her ribs to stick out, and commonly a small hollow to appear under the breast bone with each rapid chest recession. The heart beats rapidly due to the exertion of the baby.

Treatment of respiratory distress syndrome (RDS)
The baby needs oxygen. The amounts given are expressed as a percentage (%). In normal air, oxygen is present at 21 per cent. A baby with RDS may need amounts from 25 to 100 per cent. It is carefully administered and monitored.

Oxygen can be piped directly into the incubator if the baby only requires a small amount. If the baby's demand increases oxygen can be piped into a head box or plastic hood over the baby's head, or through a tiny face mask. When these methods fail to give enough oxygen, mechanical assistance is used to give oxygen directly into the lungs and to support breathing.

Continuous positive airways pressure (CPAP): This method puts a continuous controlled pressure of air and oxygen into baby's lungs. CPAP helps the baby to expand her own lungs as she breathes, so the lungs function, and oxygen is passed into the bloodstream. This method is used when the baby requires 60 per cent oxygen, or more. When CPAP fails to assist the baby's breathing, extra help is needed in the form of full artificial ventilation.

Ventilation: Oxygen and air are mixed within the ventilator and blown into the baby's lungs via a special tube which goes through the baby's mouth and rests at the top of the lungs' main air passages. The oxygen and air mixture is blown into the lungs under pressure and then a second pressure lets the lungs relax—as in normal breathing. The baby's ability to maintain a satisfactory oxygen level within her body, and thus to breathe alone, determines when the oxygen levels and pressures are reduced and when ventilation can be stopped.

Blood gases
Any baby receiving oxygen will have frequent checks made on the blood gases within the body. This is done either by continual monitoring through an oxygen-sensitive probe stuck on to the skin, or by taking at approximately four-hourly intervals a blood sample from the baby and analysing it. Blood gases show oxygen and carbon dioxide levels.

Apnoea attacks

Out of all premature babies 30 to 50 per cent will have apnoea attacks. The cause is unknown but thought to be due to the baby's 'breathing control' centre in the brain being immature. The baby simply forgets to breathe. Constant monitoring of breathing patterns by use of an apnoea alarm enables the staff to be alerted when baby stops breathing, and they can respond immediately by stimulating the baby to breathe again. Sometimes it is enough just to tap or nudge the baby's foot, or to move her, or even to tap the incubator. If baby does not respond she will be given oxygen or ventilated. It is routine to monitor all premature babies for apnoea attacks.

Why do premature babies get jaundiced?

Premature babies have a high iron level in their red blood cells. This iron is called haemoglobin—often seen written as Hb. The process to break down haemoglobin occurs at the end of each red blood cell's lifespan. Premature babies have immature red blood cells, with a short lifespan, and therefore a quick turnover of red blood cells occurs. As these blood cells are broken down, one of the substances produced is called bilirubin. This is a yellow pigment which travels to the liver via the blood, where it is normally altered by a special enzyme so it can then be excreted by the body. In the uterus the mother's enzymes take over this task—so the liver does not have to work until the baby is born. Premature babies' immature livers are slow to work initially. The enzyme needed to alter the bilirubin is only produced in small amounts. There is a rapid breakdown of red blood cells and a lot of bilirubin waiting to be altered. The liver cannot work fast enough. The unaltered yellow bilirubin stays in the bloodstream and is circulated round the body, and so the whole body looks yellow. Until the liver becomes more efficient, or until alternative treatment is given to remove the bilirubin, the baby will remain jaundiced.

The baby's skin is an orange–yellow colour and the whites of the eyes are discoloured yellow. Jaundice occurs in a third of full-term babies and most preterm babies. It makes babies sleepy, slow to feed and lethargic on handling. The staff are aware that all premature babies are at risk of developing jaundice and aim to detect it early. There is a danger that if jaundice is left undetected and untreated the levels will keep rising until there is a danger of the bilirubin damaging the brain. Nowadays this is extremely rare, as treatment and detection are simple, quick and effective.

Phototherapy treatment

The treatment for this type of jaundice is called phototherapy—which consists of a light unit being positioned over the incubator or cot and then switched on. The baby's body is bathed in light (not ultraviolet, as in sunlamps, so the baby runs no risk of getting sunburn). She is nursed naked to obtain the maximum benefit from the light—only the eyes are covered by protective eye pads or bandage, which are removed for feeding and cuddles. This light causes the bilirubin in the bloodstream to be altered, and it can then cope with getting rid of it in the motions and urine. Regular estimation of the bilirubin levels will be made by blood tests. Once the level starts to fall within safe limits the treatment is discontinued.

Exchange transfusion

Sometimes the phototherapy treatment does not reduce the bilirubin level. The treatment then is to exchange the baby's blood. This is a relatively simple procedure performed by an experienced paediatrician and nurse. A fine tube is carefully inserted into one of the baby's blood vessels. A syringe is attached and then small amounts of baby's blood are removed at a time, each time being replaced with the same amount of fresh blood from a healthy donor. Over an hour this is carefully repeated until the bilirubin is 'washed out' of baby's bloodstream. One exchange transfusion may sufficiently lower the bilirubin levels but it can be repeated several or many times. It is usually followed by phototherapy treatment.

Jaundice occurring in babies can also be caused by other

conditions. Your paediatrician will be glad to discuss matters with you if your baby is suffering from a less common sort of jaundice.

Infection

The mother's immunities are passed to the baby across the placenta during pregnancy and through breast milk after birth. The premature baby has not had time to build up her defences or to obtain all her mother's immunities. The baby has little body fat, a thin delicate skin, and is often ill—all this makes her vulnerable to infection.

If an infection is suspected, appropriate action is taken. This involves sending a specimen to the laboratory. It is examined to detect the type of infection, and tested with various antibiotic medicines to discover which antibiotic 'kills' the bacteria. A report is sent back to the SCBU and the baby is given the appropriate medicine. If it is obvious which part of the body is infected, such as a sticky eye or skin infection, then only the appropriate swabs are taken to send to the laboratory. When the source of infection is not obvious—or the baby suddenly becomes very ill—an 'infection screen' is taken. This means taking many samples and tests in order to discover where in the body system the infection is. The tests may vary slightly from different SCBUs, but will include blood tests, urine samples, swabs, and more rarely, lumbar punctures. When a lumbar puncture is performed, fluid from around the spinal cord is obtained, by an experienced doctor, by means of a fine needle and syringe. This procedure is carried out under strict sterile conditions. This fluid will show infections of the tissues around the brain.

A serious infection in one of the body systems affects a premature baby suddenly and often dramatically, causing a healthy baby to 'collapse' and become seriously ill. She will need intensive nursing and support. Once the infection is detected the baby will be isolated. Antibiotic drugs will be given to the baby—usually via a drip, or injection into the baby's muscle. Serious infections include the following:

- *Meningitis*: infection of the tissues that cover the brain and spinal cord.
- *Septicaemia*: infection in the bloodstream—therefore a generalized infection of the whole body.
- *Pneumonia*: infection within the lungs—this causes breathing problems. The baby can be born with pneumonia if prolonged rupture of the membranes had occurred, or can acquire it after birth.
- *Diarrhoea and vomiting*: infection in the intestines causing serious illness in the baby. If several babies catch this type of infection, units have to close down until the infection clears.

In some units all the babies are given antibiotics routinely to help prevent serious infections.

Anaemia

Premature babies have a tendency to become anaemic because they are often subjected to many blood tests. They have no iron stores in their bodies and extra iron cannot be given in the form of medicine because the baby's immature system can not efficiently metabolize and therefore absorb the iron. So haemoglobin levels fall, and the baby, having no iron stores to fall back on, becomes anaemic. As it is common for premature babies to become anaemic, it is routine to give 'top-up transfusions' of fresh donor blood through a drip. Some units keep careful records of blood samples, replacing the blood with a 'top-up' when a certain amount has been removed. Top-up transfusions can be given several times during baby's hospital stay.

Heart murmur

A heart murmur is heard by the paediatrician when he listens to the heartbeat through a stethoscope. A murmur is a turbulent flow of blood heard in the heart. This does occur frequently in premature babies and is usually caused by a temporary 'flap' in the heart failing to close properly. Very often it is of no significance, the baby remains well and the murmur disappears in time as the heart matures and the flap closes. A careful follow-up of the baby at clinic will be done until the murmur has gone. Occasionally the baby may be given drugs to help close this 'flap' in the heart, but this depends upon the paediatrician and how bad the murmur is. Many babies are routinely referred to a cardiac (heart) specialist.

The premature baby's brain

The brain continues to develop and grow more or less as it would if the baby was still inside the mother, although it does have to withstand more complex demands in learning to adjust to the outside world before full maturity. Ultrasound brain scans are performed routinely in many SCBUs to check that all is well. The scan will show the size of the brain and if there is any excess fluid. It will also show any bleeding within the brain, so scans are performed to check on any suspected brain haemorrhage—in premature babies this is fairly common and not necessarily of any significance. It may be slight or extensive, and is more often found in babies who have had oxygen therapy.

The brain is made up of two halves, called ventricles, and has a very rich blood supply to keep it well supplied with oxygen. The 'floor' of the two ventricles have many tiny blood vessels, like miniature capillaries, which can burst, causing a small leakage of blood. This is called an intraventricular haemorrhage (IVH). Often this occurs and heals over undetected, but occasionally it can be of a more serious and damaging nature. Some units give vitamin E, aiming to reduce the incidence of extensive brain haemorrhage. The paediatrician will explain more fully and specifically the implications of any IVH if this applies to your baby. *It is important to note that IVH is not necessarily an indication that the brain will be damaged.*

Brain damage

The baby's condition is continually assessed during labour,

so that any signs of distress can be detected early, and prompt medical action taken to prevent brain damage. Delivery in hospital is therefore very important for premature babies. Thankfully, due to the vigilance and care of obstetricians and midwives at antenatal clinics, the vast majority of preterm labours take place in hospital. High-risk patients are often admitted early to ensure a hospital delivery. This is why only a very tiny minority of premature babies suffers brain damage. The risk is there, but medical procedures reduce the risk greatly, and very, very few babies suffer from brain damage.

Transferring the ill baby

When a baby becomes seriously ill and is referred to an intensive care unit it is frequently necessary to transfer the baby. This is usually to a neonatal intensive care unit (NICU) in the nearest large city. The receiving hospital sends a paediatrician and nursing staff from the unit in a specially equipped ambulance to collect the baby. This team should meet the parents to explain what is happening and invite them to come to the unit as soon as possible. Mothers and fathers should be able to accompany their baby.

The baby will travel in a transport incubator, with a built-in mechanical ventilator and other monitoring devices. It works off its own rechargeable battery and is secured inside the back of the ambulance. The paediatrician and nurse will stabilize the baby's condition if necessary on the SCBU, collect all the relevant notes, tests, etc. and then continue to give the baby the care she needs during the journey. This could include ventilation, full monitoring and emergency procedures.

If your baby is transferred for intensive care it can be reassuring to know that she will return to your local SCBU once she is better and the intensive care is no longer needed.

If you cannot travel with your baby in the ambulance, you may like to make your own arrangements to be near the baby in her new hospital.

Baptism

It is a normal procedure in all SCBUs and NICUs to suggest that the baby should be baptized when she is seriously ill. It can be very comforting and reassuring to have your baby baptized. Your own minister, or more usually the hospital's own chaplain, will perform the baptism. The short service can be performed anywhere on the unit, respectfully, quietly and with reverence.

You will receive a small certificate of baptism. Later on you may wish to have a more celebratory christening when all is well and baby is safely home. Most denominations will perform a special service.

If you do not have your baby baptized and the baby dies, baptism can be performed up to an hour following death.

Losing a baby

I was frightened to love her too much in case she died.

It is quite a normal feeling, not wanting to let yourself love the baby, and surely a thought that must pass through the minds of most parents. It is hard to allow love to develop when your baby is seriously ill and fighting for life, it is harder still when you know the baby is dying. But no matter how short a time the baby lives, she is here now and will benefit from your love and affection. Do try to let your loving instincts override the fear of death, get to know your baby, and your memories of her will be memories of a real little person who received all the love her parents could possibly give.

After the baby has died

You will feel numb and shocked and may wish to be alone with your partner or someone close to you in a room with the baby. This is not morbid; it is a natural desire to be alone with your baby, to look at her in peace. The nurses will stay with you if this makes you feel happier. All the tubes, wires and intensive care trappings will be removed and the baby laid to rest. You may be comforted by some religious support—this is available and hospital chaplains are experienced in helping bereaved parents.

We found that parents who did not see or hold their babies regretted it in the weeks to come and encouraged parents in similar circumstances to do so. It helps so much, providing memories of your baby as a real little person who did exist and live for a brief time.

Some parents, however, simply can not bring themselves to see their dying or dead baby. While we would advise any parents who are *uncertain* whether to see their dead infant or not, to take courage and go, we would certainly *not* suggest that parents *ought* to go. You must try to decide for yourselves what to do—it is entirely natural and understandable not to want to see a baby who has died. At the same time, it is normal, and not morbid, to want to see your baby for the last time. Do what your instincts tell you—and rest assured that *your* decision is the right one.

Medical terms

When your baby is in special care or intensive care, you may be worried about the medical terms you hear. Our advice is that you talk with the staff as fully as you can, so that any medical terminology is clearly explained to you. A brief glossary of terms is given on page 105.

FIVE

Feeding

During the 40 weeks when a baby is inside her mother's uterus, she is receiving all the nutrition she needs from her mother. At around 40 weeks, however, labour begins and the baby is born into the outside world where she must begin to take in nourishment by herself. Normally, of course, the healthy newborn baby will be put to the breast or offered a bottle of baby milk, and milk feeding is established within a few days. The full-term baby is ready for her milk—her digestive system is mature, and she quickly learns how to suck. She can digest her milk and she will thrive and grow.

But, if a baby is born prematurely she may be more difficult to feed. Her tiny body may not have matured enough for normal digestion to take place efficiently, so that she cannot tolerate milk. She may be too ill to feed, or she may be too tired or unable to suck. Your baby's ability to take milk from breast or bottle will depend largely on how premature she was, or how ill she is.

Feeding before milk

The newly born premature baby will be assessed by a paediatrician who will then decide how to provide her with the nutrients she needs. Normally this will entail tube feeding with milk, but in some cases milk will not be given. The medical team may give a sick or very premature baby a dextrose solution, a colourless water and sugar fluid, usually given by drip into a scalp vein. This solution prevents the baby from dehydrating and gives her a little energy. Dextrose may be given for several days, depending on how sick the baby is.

Total parenteral nutrition

Very premature babies (25 or 26 weeks) and those babies who are very ill may be given total parenteral nutrition. This is a more complete solution of nutrients given by drip. Total parenteral nutrition will be given until the paediatrician judges that the baby can tolerate tiny amounts of milk. Each baby is a unique case, and there are no set rules for feeding. The doctors and nurses will design a planned scheme of nutrition especially for your baby, and in doing this they will always take into account the prematurity and the health of your baby before deciding how she should be nourished.

Tube feeding

When the baby's condition stabilizes, the next step is to offer her a little milk, usually by tube. This is because premature babies cannot usually suck and swallow effectively until around 34 weeks' gestation. Tube feeding enables them to take in milk without any effort, and thus they are receiving the nourishment they need while conserving their energy. A trained nurse will put the feeding tube in place. A *nasogastric* tube is a very thin fine hollow tube which is passed through the baby's nostril down into her stomach. It is then secured, usually by a piece of adhesive tape on her nose or cheek. The tube is left in place and changed every day, or more if necessary. Occasionally a baby will pull at her tube, but this is nothing to worry about. *A nasojejunal* tube is a fine hollow tube which passes through the nostril into the stomach, and then beyond the stomach into the first section of the intestine—the jejunum. This avoids distending a baby's stomach, and is used often on very sick or very premature babies.

Milk is given to the baby via the tube, either by continuous feeding with an electric pump, when tiny amounts of milk are administered automatically at very frequent intervals, or by intermittent feeding. In this method, a small sterile syringe container is attached to the end of the tube, filled with exactly the right amount of milk, and then held up above the baby's head. The milk then falls gradually by gravity into her stomach. How much milk to give is determined by the baby's health, weight and maturity, and the intervals between feeds will also be decided, taking these factors into consideration. Before each feed, a little food is withdrawn by the nurse from the baby's stomach, using a suction syringe. The small amount of food is tested, and this will tell the nurse whether or not the tube is still positioned in the stomach and whether the milk is being digested.

Your baby could be tube-fed for several days or even weeks, again depending on her immaturity and health. A good SCBU will encourage parents to participate in tube-feeding; the nurses will show you the correct way, and will supervise while you hold your baby and her tube of milk.

Your baby's nutritional needs

Premature babies have special nutritional needs which differ from those of full-term babies. Basically, they need more minerals and trace elements such as sodium, phosphorus and calcium, because these are normally laid down in the baby's body during the last two months of gestation. These last, vital weeks, when stores of energy and minerals are accumulated in the baby's body, are missed when she is born too soon. Therefore, premature babies are in a precarious state, nutritionally speaking. Their reserves are low, their metabolic rate is high, they need and use more energy to keep warm and they need more protein for growth than full-term infants. At the same time, their immature kidneys and digestive systems are less able to absorb nutrients and excrete waste. Breast milk and ordinary formulas will nourish the baby, but relatively large quantities are needed for normal growth and development to occur. The problem then is to try to feed the premature baby with an easily digested milk which will enable the baby to grow at roughly the same rate as if she had still been in the womb, will supply her with the missing stores, and will give her enough calories for her energy expenditure.

Ordinary baby formula
Ordinary powdered milks are, of course, lacking in these extra nutrients and energy, but they may be suitable if your baby was only a week or two premature and if you intend to bottle feed.

Low birth-weight formula
These powdered milks have been specially prepared for small and premature babies. They contain a more suitable compound of elements, proteins, and other nutrients for a baby who has missed the last weeks of her gestation. They have been formulated to an excellent standard and premature babies fed with these low birth-weight milks have thrived and put on much-needed weight in the early days, while only needing relatively small quantities of this milk. Thus, premature babies, especially those born very early, say 26 to 32 weeks, get more benefit from these special milks than from ordinary powdered milks. These low birth-weight milks are normally only used in hospitals and for only short periods. They, of course, lack protective immunizing factors contained in breast milk.

Breast milk

Breast milk is especially valuable for tiny premature babies, although very small immature babies under 30 weeks' gestation may need special high energy supplements and extra minerals and vitamins. It is much easier for a premature baby to digest than any powdered formula, and it protects premature babies from infection, because it contains substances which act to prevent dangerous bacteria from flourishing in the baby's intestines. Premature babies are very susceptible to infection, and breast milk is the best possible safeguard against it. As well as all this, breast milk contains exactly the right balance of nutrients for your baby to grow and develop. Recently, much evidence has accumulated which shows that the very best milk for premature babies is human milk, although extra energy and minerals may need to be added.[13] Studies have shown that breast milk given to premature babies produces a growth curve which closely follows that of the intra-uterine growth curve. It has been demonstrated that the colostrum —the rich, creamy milk secreted by a mother during the first days of milk production—of mothers who deliver premature babies differs from normal. Amazingly, it contains more of the trace minerals[14] which the baby needs, but which she lacks because she has missed out on the last vital gestational weeks when these mineral stores are laid down. Recent research has shown too that breast milk from mothers of premature babies is higher in protein—to help the baby grow and develop—than breast milk from mothers of full-term babies.

It is thought that babies given breast milk soon after birth suffer from fewer convulsions and apnoeic attacks (periods of stopping breathing).

When your baby is ready to take milk, the medical team will discuss with you which milk she should have. Feeding a premature baby is largely a matter of trial and error. If it is found that your baby needs extra help to put on weight she will be given extra calories to supplement your breast milk. She may be given a low birth-weight formula as well as your milk, or she may be given special high-calorie solutions. Therefore, if you have decided that your baby should have breast milk, and the paediatrician wants to give her a low birth-weight formula as well, try not to feel disappointed. The formula will give her the extra calories she needs to grow a little stronger, and she need not stop taking your precious, irreplaceable breast milk.

Breastfeeding your premature baby

If you decide to breastfeed your baby, you are giving her the best opportunity to thrive and you are providing her immature, weak body with protection against dangerous bacteria. You are also giving her a unique food which no-one else can provide, and when you actually begin to suckle her you will be forming the roots of a solid, loving relationship which will stand steady long after she is weaned. Knowing that you are doing so much for your baby will help you overcome any difficulties and hurdles on the way to establishing total breastfeeding. Many mothers in our sample said that breastfeeding was a wonderful, positive way to bridge the initial separation.

> Expressing milk became my emotional support—it proved that I had a baby who existed, and it gave me a routine and a feeling that I was doing all I could.

Expressing breast milk

Immediately after delivery, you may be able to hold your baby for a very short while. If she is very premature it will not be possible for her to suckle at this special time, straight after the birth. Try not to feel disappointed. Your baby's first need is prompt medical attention because she may have breathing difficulties and she must be kept warm. Instead, send a message to the SCBU that you plan to breastfeed your baby, and if possible you would like her to have EBM (expressed breast milk) only. When the nurses learn that you are keen to try breastfeeding you will be shown how to express your breast milk. As we have seen, your baby may be too immature or too ill to suck normally from your breast, but if you do not express milk yourself, your milk will not be stimulated and your supply will gradually dwindle so that there will be no milk when your baby is ready to suckle. Expressing is the *only* way to initiate and build up a good supply of breast milk which can be fed to your baby as soon as she is ready, via a tube. When she is mature enough to try suckling, you will have a good supply ready for her.

The hospital staff will show you how to express milk, and should do all they can to help you establish a good supply of breast milk. You should begin to express your breast milk as soon as possible after the birth. If you are very ill following delivery this may delay starting, but need not deter you. You can still express as soon as you are able, making it a priority in your routine, both in the early days in hospital and when you are discharged, to express frequently. This is the only way to succeed.

There are several ways to express breast milk, the most efficient being an electric breast pump.

Electric breast pump

This is a machine small enough to fit on a table top which works very effectively to simulate the sucking action of a baby. It is the most effective way to express milk, if done properly. You will be shown how to sit comfortably in front of the machine and try, above all, to relax. Tension and stress tend to inhibit milk production, and although it is difficult when you are worried about your baby, you must try to relax. Try closing your eyes and breathing deeply—feel your muscles relaxing as you sit quietly and at ease in a comfortable chair.

Briefly, the machine works like this. You attach a small, sterile glass bottle or plastic container to the machine using a length of sterile tube. To the bottle or container you attach a sterile breast cup, which looks like a small plastic or glass funnel. (All this equipment must be stored in a sterilizing solution, and you must take great care to have clean hands and nipples.) The funnel is then placed over your nipple and the machine switched on. For your first attempts you will be asked to use the electric pump on its lowest suction strength, and for only a minute or two on each side. When the machine is switched on, it creates an intermittent vacuum in the thin tube attached to your collecting bottle and this causes a sucking action at your nipple. The machine times itself to suck steadily on and off, rhythmically, like a baby. This sucking action stimulates the milk glands to produce milk and gradually the first milk, in the form of colostrum, will begin to appear. At your first try you may not get any colostrum, but if you keep using the pump regularly you should succeed. Any colostrum you manage to express, however meagre the quantity—and at best it will only be a few millilitres in the bottom of the container—is worth more than its weight in gold; it can even be frozen for later use if the baby is too sick or immature.

> On the third day I began to regularly express breast milk. At last I had *something* to do for my son. On his chart in the evening was the comment—'Fresh EBM given by tube'. Although I saw that it was only 5 ml, it gave me a very satisfying feeling.

You will be able to use the machine at a higher suction level as time goes on. A lever setting of medium or high gives a stronger suck, and thus more stimulation to produce milk.

A most valuable source of help and advice is the National Childbirth Trust. They publish two excellent leaflets.[15] Your local NCT branch will be very helpful. Contact them for a discussion with the local breastfeeding counsellor; she will know all about pumps and expressing milk, and her advice and tips will be very useful. She will be happy to advise you, even if you are not a member of the NCT. She will also be able to arrange for you to hire an electric breast pump to take home with you so that you can express milk properly and regularly for as long as you need to. The cost varies from area to area.

Make sure that the breast pump is working properly. This may not be easy, since not many people know how to maintain and service them, but it is important.

We have shown the importance of relaxing while expressing. Many mothers found that a photo of baby, propped up by the pump, helped them to 'let down' their milk.

Try to imagine that you are actually feeding your baby. Listen to some music, read a magazine, or watch television —in short, make yourself comfortable. Your milk will let down more easily and in greater quantities. You will have a greater chance of success if you express little and often. Five minutes expressing each side, six times a day, will be more successful than ten minutes, four times a day. Try to organize your own routine, when you are at home, around the other important factors of your day. Other children's needs may alter your breast pump schedule—try to fit the 'feeds' in as best you can.

You need extra rest at this time—impossible though it sounds! With visits to the hospital, and coping with normal life, you may not have the time to put up your feet for a few minutes, but it really is *very* important. Ask for help with housework, shopping, and the children, and remember that a couple of 30-minute rests each day really does increase your milk production. Keep your meals simple and nutritious, and remember that a breastfeeding mother needs an extra 500 calories a day. A drink at expressing times will keep up your vital fluid intake, and brewers' yeast tablets from the chemist may be helpful.

How much milk will I manage to express?

Your premature baby's needs will be assessed by the paediatrician or the sister on the unit. However, breast milk is not regulated by computer! You cannot possibly express the exact amount of milk your baby needs at each session. What happens is that your breasts will supply milk erratically. You will find that normally you will be able to express a lot of milk first thing in the morning, and only a little in the evening. Therefore, if the total milk production over 24 hours, or better still, a week, is added up you will have a much better guide as to how much milk you are making, on average. The first and most important thing to stress about how much milk you make is that it doesn't really matter. Your primary aim while using a breast pump is to build up and maintain a flow of milk, no matter how little you manage to express at each session. The best form of stimulation is a baby at your nipple, but many mothers are unable to put their baby to the breast for *at least* a week or so. The baby may be too weak, immature, or ill to suck. These mothers have to make do with the next best thing, a breast pump. Using a pump *often* will stimulate your supply ready for when your baby can suckle.

The collecting bottles with an electric breast pump can usually hold 100 ml of milk, although the modern Egnell pump provides a plastic container which holds about 200 ml. If you manage 100 ml at a typical pumping session, you will be doing very well indeed; 50 or 60 ml is a more average, perfectly acceptable amount, and less than this is a comparatively small amount but still adequate. If you are only making a very little milk, *do not* give up. The SCBU staff will receive it gratefully and your baby will benefit tremendously, even if she has to have extra top-ups of donated or formula milk. If you are worried about this, talk it over with your SCBU sister. She will be very happy to discuss it with you.

If you find that you can only express a very small amount of milk, say 10 or 20 ml you are probably not getting a let-down reflex. This means that you are getting foremilk, but that your hindmilk—the store of milk in the ducts deep inside your breasts—is not being let down; the muscles around the milk ducts are not contracting. You can usually tell if you are experiencing a 'let-down'. It can be felt as a sort of slight ache in the breasts lasting for a second or two. Some women describe it as a 'tingling' or 'fizzing' sensation. It can be slight or strong, like all muscle contractions.

If you are not experiencing a let-down, try to relax, and follow our suggestions to read, watch TV, listen to music, have a drink, eat a snack, and generally adopt a casual, less tense attitude to the breast pump. If these tips don't work, ask your general practitioner for a Syntocinon spray. This will stimulate a let-down reflex. Once you have felt the let-down, you will find that the milk will flow readily.

If you get the chance to cuddle or hold your baby during a visit, this will help to stimulate your milk production. Talking to her and stroking her soft body will help to make you feel emotionally close to her, and your maternal feelings will increase. Many mothers in our sample found this to be a vital part of expressing milk.

Sometimes, mothers find that they suffer from sore nipples and painful breast engorgement, just as if they were feeding their baby. If this happens, ask the nurse, health visitor, midwife, or doctor for advice. Both conditions clear up quickly and do not mean that you have to stop expressing.

Don't worry if it takes you some time to establish effective breast milk expression—at least seven days, and up to three weeks. Don't give up hope.

If, despite all your efforts and determination, you find that you really are unable to express milk you must not be despondent. Only 49 per cent of mothers in our sample managed to establish breastfeeding. It really is not the easiest thing to accomplish, and your baby will be given the best possible alternative—probably a low birth-weight formula, and later one of the many excellent baby milks available.

Syringe-type pumps

These are fairly efficient, though not so good as electric pumps. They look like a large test tube, and they work on the syringe principle. By working the outer cylinder in and out, while the breast cup is placed over the nipple area, a rhythmical movement can be achieved which is similar to a baby's sucking action. The expressed milk collects in the inner cylinder, which can be used as a bottle if necessary by attaching a teat to it. The advantage of a syringe-type pump is that it is cheap to buy (from a chemist), and it has a gentler action than an electric pump. It can be controlled directly by the user. You will need to be shown how to operate the pump properly, so seek advice. Hospitals will often lend you one free of charge, but if you can afford to buy one, they are very cheap and readily available from large chemists.

Bulb pumps

These look like a glass bulb with a cup shape at one end and a flexible rubber or plastic ball at the other. They are sometimes called breast relievers, and can be bought cheaply at most chemists. The cup shape fits over the nipple and by squeezing and releasing the flexible ball, milk can be coaxed out of the breast. However, these pumps are not usually very effective, though a few mothers have found them useful.

Hand expressing

Hand expressing is the cheapest method of all since it requires no special equipment. Not everyone finds it easy to acquire the knack of expressing by hand, but once you can do it it is very useful for expressing small amounts of milk. You may find that expressing a little excess milk by hand relieves breast engorgement and it is useful when your nipples are cracked or very sore. Again, the best way to learn is from a midwife or from a mother who is breastfeeding and who can demonstrate the action.

Hygiene: Milk is an ideal environment for bacteria to thrive and multiply, so it is most important to observe good standards of hygiene when you are expressing milk. Make sure you always wash your hands before expressing, and that your nipples are clean. You will be shown how to wash thoroughly and sterilize any parts of the pumps which have been in contact with milk. It is a good idea to keep a fresh sterilizing solution handy, so that all the bits and pieces can be put straight in the solution after washing. This procedure also applies to the small bottles or plastic containers given to you by the hospital for your collected milk. Your expressed milk should be transferred immediately from the collecting vessel to the bottle or container supplied. These bottles might be specially sterilized and sealed in plastic bags ready for your use. If you do re-use any bottles, you must soak them in sterilizing solution first. Breast milk put into bottles must be placed well inside the refrigerator and used or taken to the SCBU as soon as possible, preferably within 48 hours—clearly labelled with your name, and the date and exact time of expressing. Never mix newly expressed milk with older milk. It is worthwhile considering freezing your milk if this method suits you, and special plastic containers can be used and are provided by some hospitals. Basically, you must remember to observe hygiene, to seal the plastic bottles properly before placing them in a freezer, and to ensure that the milk is frozen quickly, on fast-freeze if you can, to a temperature of at least −18° C. Care must be taken when thawing out milk. It is best thawed in the fridge, and then used as soon as possible. Freezers are a useful way of extending the storage life of breast milk—but they are not totally sterile.

Am I tempting fate?

It is very common for mothers to feel uneasy about expressing breast milk in the early days after delivery. If the baby is well and only four weeks premature it seems only natural to assume that she will survive and begin breast-feeding after a few days. But if your baby is only 32 weeks' gestation—or even younger—you may be so worried for her survival that expressing breast milk seems futile. This is a normal reaction, and some mothers are so completely unable to overcome the severe stress of the situation that they do not even consider expressing their breast milk.

You should realize that by expressing breast milk for your baby, you are actively increasing her chances of survival, and you are giving her the best milk she can possibly have during her first immature weeks. Your milk is unique, irreplaceable, and very, very precious—being extremely rich in protective antibodies and nutrients. Indeed, one of the reasons why premature babies nowadays have an excellent chance of survival and normal development is that we understand much more about their nutritional needs.

Establishing breastfeeding

As we have seen, the first step is to build up and maintain a flow of breast milk, using a good breast pump. You may have to express your milk for a week or two, or perhaps several weeks, or even two or three months, depending on how premature your baby is.

Premature babies can usually suck from around 34 weeks, but the paediatrician and the nursing staff should be watching your baby for signs of the rooting instinct and lip and tongue movements. When they feel that your baby can try sucking for herself, they should discuss this with you.

Bottles

Many units have a 'bottle first' policy. A little EBM (expressed breast milk) is put into a feeding bottle, and your baby is encouraged to suck from the teat. The reasoning here is that premature babies are weak and tire very easily when they are sucking. They are using up precious energy to suck, and even a minute's sucking can make a tiny premature baby very sleepy indeed. It is much easier for her to suck milk from a bottle. She does not have to work so hard to get her milk, and so she will be satisfied earlier, and with less expended effort. She is using few calories and therefore she will gain weight more readily. However, some units do not always use bottles first. The drawback, it is argued, is that baby will become used to a teat and will subsequently reject the nipple. Also, the sucking action of a baby feeding from a bottle teat is different from when she feeds from the breast. This can cause difficulty when the mother actually begins to breastfeed.

The baby, if she accepts the nipple in the first place, will not be able to suck efficiently on this 'new' shape. She will have to relearn her sucking technique. She may become frustrated, and exhausted, and her mother upset and disappointed that she hasn't succeeded. If the sister in your unit has specified that a bottle should be used at first with your baby, talk it over with her until you are satisfied in your own mind. Remember that the staff only want the best for your baby, and that they are acting in *her* interests. Remember too that she is *your* baby! Work together with the staff to formulate the best plan for establishing breastfeeding.

If your baby is given bottles of your expressed breast milk it is worth trying to obtain and use a bottle teat which is shaped more like a nipple. These are often available from the NCT's local breastfeeding counsellor, and from large chemists. Ask the hospital if your natural-shaped teats can be used with your baby's bottles.

When it is clear that your baby can take milk from a bottle, she will gradually be given more and more bottle feeds until her feeding tube can eventually be removed. During this time you will be able to try your first breast feed.

She may now be taking milk at, say, three-hourly intervals, instead of one or two hourly, because she is a little stronger, more mature, and bigger. Her stomach can hold more milk, she can take more milk at one feed. Each baby's feeding schedule is unique, but a typical schedule will be to build up gradually to alternate bottle and breast feeds. Then you will be able to breastfeed her more frequently, until she is feeding from you every time.

> Every time we visited I put him to the breast and at ten days he sucked for the first time. From then on it was fairly plain sailing.

The first breastfeed

When this long-awaited day comes, you must temper your

excitement with a little sensible calm relaxation. Your baby will probably be very sleepy and will have to learn how to suck from your nipple. Don't expect too much from the first feed. Above all, try to relax, talk gently to your baby, and concentrate on loving her. Try not to be nervous, she will be sensitive to your mood and will pick up your tension. Be positive, calm, gentle, and quietly confident. Sit comfortably in a quiet corner, and relax. The nurse will help your baby to latch on to your breast; remember that she is experienced and can help you overcome any initial difficulties. If you are a first-time mother, and breastfeeding is new to you, be guided by the nurse. She will help you and can be a great support to you during your 'learning' time. Once baby has 'latched on' to your nipple, she will begin to suck. She may suck only for a minute or two before falling asleep. This first attempt at breastfeeding will be largely a matter of trial and error for both you and baby, but with patience and support from an experienced nurse, a few relaxed sessions should be enough to give the baby the general idea. If she doesn't seem interested the first time, she may do better the next time—or the next. Soon you will both be more confident, and breastfeeding will come more easily.

> I was very upset that he couldn't suck and feed-times became rather stressful. It was rather a shock to discover that breastfeeding did not come naturally.

Useful tips for breastfeeding

Each mother-baby partnership is unique, and only the three of you—mother, baby and experienced nurse or helper—can work out the best approach to success. However, here are a few tips.

- Brush your baby's cheek with your nipple. Her head will turn towards it and her mouth will open.

- Make sure the baby gets more than just the tip of the nipple in her mouth. Her mouth should cover the areola as well. Breastfeeding a premature baby in the early days can be more difficult than breastfeeding a full-term baby, not only because she is sleepy, weak and immature, and possibly used to a bottle teat, but also because of the actual physical mechanics of sucking. The baby's mouth is very small compared to that of a full-term baby, so the baby may produce 'nipple traction', making breastfeeding uncomfortable for the mother. In other words, more parts of the baby's mouth are rubbing on the nipple, so that sore nipples are fairly common. The answer is to make sure that the baby opens her mouth wide to fix properly on to the areola. A skilled midwife will help you to do this.

- Be prepared to spend a lot of time with your baby during these early days.

- Try expressing a little milk into the baby's mouth, or on to the end of your nipple. This may stimulate her.

- Expressing a little milk beforehand is useful if your breasts are very full, because your baby will not be able to latch on to an overfull, engorged breast. Expressing makes the nipple easier to grasp.

- Use a Syntocinon nasal spray to stimulate a let-down.

- Nipple shields can help if your nipples are flat, or sore. The best kind is made completely of rubber, shaped like a Mexican hat, and is often known as the natural nursing nipple shield. Your NCT counsellor will have one available.

- To wake a sleepy baby for her feed, unwrap her a little so that she is still warm but not so securely wrapped. Tickle her toes or her arm or leg, or lift her up over your shoulder. Talk to her, play some music to her, perhaps a musical mobile or toy.

- It has been found that premature babies' intake of milk during feeding is increased when little social interaction takes place.[16] Save the talking for another time.

With practice and patience, you should become more confident and you will both begin to succeed, although your baby may still tire easily and may still need feeding very often. As your breastfeeding sessions increase and your baby grows stronger, you will be well on the way to success.

Expressing

Even though you have established breastfeeding successfully, you should still continue to use the breast pump. Carry on expressing normally and regularly, at first, and as your baby takes more and more feeds from you, you can begin to lessen the pumping sessions. Don't hurry to do this, though, or your milk supply will dwindle through lack of stimulation.

Weight gain

Once the baby's condition stabilizes, her feeding and weight is closely monitored. The SCBU staff want to see a regular weight gain. This shows that the baby is digesting her milk and is thriving. If feed charts and weighing sessions become unbearably significant, overshadowing your entire life, do not despair! The preoccupation with weight gain is purely for the benefit of your baby. If she gains weight regularly and feeds properly, she is ready to go home.

Some mothers viewed weighing sessions with great trepidation, as though they were somehow tests of personal achievement, and indeed some SCBUs seem inadvertently to exaggerate the situation by weighing the babies with great ceremony and comment. Good units will reassure parents that regular weight checks are only done as a guide to the baby's well-being.

Establishing bottle feeding

If you do not intend to breastfeed your baby, or if for some reason you are unable to establish breastfeeding, then she will be very gradually weaned from feeding tube to bottle. When the SCBU staff feel that she is able to try sucking from a teat, a bottle feed will be tried.

Which milk?

There are several excellent baby milks available which are designed specially for low birth-weight and premature babies, containing all the nutrients your baby needs. They are only used in hospitals, although if your baby is discharged fairly early because she is fit and well, the SCBU may give you a supply of low birth-weight formula to continue at home for a while. However, if your baby was a fairly late gestation, say over 34 weeks, she may be given an ordinary formula straight away. These are also excellent and are usually supplied to hospitals ready mixed in small bottles. Each SCBU usually has its favoured formula milks.

Teats

The special care unit will have soft teats especially designed for newborn babies. They are prepacked and a new one is used at every feed. It is attached straight on to the small bottle of prepared milk, so that the baby has a sterile germ-free teat at every feed. Some SCBUs have their own supply of ordinary teats which they keep sterilized.

If your baby's mouth is so small that she seems not able to cope with a normal teat, it is well worth trying another type, with a different shape. NUK teats are shaped more like a nipple as are several other brands currently available; incidentally, NUK dummies are available too, both from the NCT. A Playtex Nurser is also an alternative shaped teat which your baby might find easier to grasp; it is available from large chemists.

The first feed

Ask if you can give your baby her very first bottle feed—it is important for you both. You will get to know your baby best by feeding and caring for her and she will benefit from having individualized care—that is, her feeds and daily care from the same person each time. If you participate as much as possible, by giving her as many bottle feeds as you can, you will have the best opportunity to form the basis of a close loving relationship.

Your baby will be wrapped up warmly and given to you. Sit comfortably, and try to be calm and relaxed. Talk to her, and if she is sleepy, follow our tips for waking her. Loosen her blankets, and stroke her face, arms or toes. Change her position, hold her upright, and play a musical toy. When she opens her eyes and becomes alert, you can try the feed.

Hold her close, and very gently touch her cheek or lips with the teat. Letting a drop of milk fall into her mouth may stimulate her. The midwife should be with you so that her experience and your love will be the best combination at this special moment. Be guided by the midwife and ask questions if you are worried. She will be very happy to help you. Don't worry if your baby doesn't seem interested. She may do better next time. If she grasps the teat and sucks, well and good, but if not, she will at least be learning the feel and smell of the teat and milk. A minute or two of sucking may make her very tired, so again don't worry if she falls asleep. With patience you, better than anyone, can help your baby to get the idea of feeding from a bottle.

Rooming in

When it is clear that your baby is fit, gaining weight regularly, and feeding well, she is ready to go home. However, the SCBU staff will want to ensure that you are quite confident about feeding and caring for her. If you are already making use of the SCBU's residential facilities, this confidence will grow gradually because you will have spent most of your time with your baby. If you have been unable to stay in the SCBU, then you will have been visiting regularly. Most units ask you to come and stay, using one of their specially provided bedrooms, for two or more days just before your baby is ready for discharge. Be prepared for this, because it is a valuable experience for you both.

SIX

Going Home

When it becomes apparent that your baby is beginning to thrive, the SCBU staff will have a fairly good idea of when she will be able to go home. Some units have a goal weight, which may be around 5 lbs (2270 g), but it is more usual not to wait for any 'magic' weight, but to discharge the baby when she is fit, feeding well, putting on weight regularly, and able to maintain her own body temperature. The last weeks before discharge can seem terribly long and frustrating, but if you stay in communication with the staff, you will find that they too are eager for the baby to go home—another one of their success stories! You have all worked hard for your baby's life, and when the time comes for her to be safely discharged, you will all rejoice, parents and medical team alike. The paediatrician is more likely to discharge a baby early if he knows that you are caring, conscientious, loving parents. It is felt that in these circumstances an early discharge is beneficial for parents and baby—fewer re-admissions occur, and breastfeeding is more likely to be successful.

When the staff are more confident about your baby, they will talk with you about her discharge. It may be in several weeks, or even several days. They cannot give a definite date because so much depends on the baby, but you can start to prepare for her homecoming. Some parents were wary of buying baby clothes and equipment too soon, and naturally so, but try to be positive as soon as you can. Leaving everything until the last minute leads to flustered, overtired parents—not an ideal state of mind for bringing your baby home.

Clothing and equipment

Most of the baby equipment you will need is the same as for

a full-term baby. If you are unsure about the basic necessities, get advice from your health visitor, midwife, NCT branch, or a good babycare manual (we recommend Penelope Leach's *Baby and Child*). However, there are things to look out for.

Clothes

Back at home, I was left with the job of finding something small enough for Katherine to wear. Everything looked so ridiculous.

First-size baby clothes will probably be far too big for your premature baby. A 'newborn' size babystretch suit, size 60 cm, will fit your baby from about 6½ lbs (2940 g), as a rough guide. So if your baby is one of the thousands of low birth-weight babies coming home at around 4 lbs (1814 g), a 60 cm-size babystretch suit will be far too big, and so will all normal first-size vests, hats, etc.—'First size woolly vests came down to his ankles! Everything seems geared for chubby babies.'

The only mothers who seemed happy with the normal first-size clothes were those whose babies had been discharged at 5½ lbs (2490 g) or over. We also found that parents whose babies did wear special low birth weight clothes, continued to use them for many weeks. So if your baby weighs around 4 lbs (1814 g) on discharge, consider buying three plain stretch suits, at least, from a special low birth-weight range of clothes. Friends and relatives may also be persuaded to buy small gifts of low birth-weight clothing. Make sure that the stretch suits can be machine-washed, unless you don't mind handwashing, and that you do not use them when your baby has obviously outgrown them. Her toes may be constricted in a too tight suit. If you are considering buying other clothes, such as tiny dungarees, tops and vests from a low birth-weight range, make sure that they are warm, preferably machine-washable, and *wearable*. Pretty dresses and romper suits are, in our opinion, not essential. We recommend three stretch suits, three vests and possibly a fleecy sleepsuit. These will fit properly, keep her warm, and look attractive. Suppliers' addresses can be found on page 111.

- Remember that *some* ordinary baby clothes may be suitable for your tiny baby. Shop around—if you have time!—because some parents found tiny clothes available from markets, and that chain-stores' own-name brands tend to be smaller.

- Anything *ribbed* or very stretchy will be a better fit. Parents found that ribbed jumpers etc. were quite suitable for their tiny babies.

- Your baby will need clothes mainly for *warmth*. A good, well-fitting (not tight) babygrow and vest will keep her warmer than excessively baggy, ill-fitting clothes. For the best body insulation, buy good vests, good babygrows, a fleecy sleepsuit if possible, and plenty of well-fitting *warm* bonnets. Hands and feet get cold quickly, so mittens are invaluable, as are bootees, particularly when worn *over* babygrows.

- You and your friends and relatives may, of course, consider sewing and knitting small clothes for your baby. Doll-sized patterns may be useful, especially for knitwear, but make sure that the clothes have enough fasteners, and that they are suitable for babies. (Dolls' clothes *bought* from toy shops are *not* recommended, as they are not suitable for babies, in many ways.) Sirdar do knitting patterns in a 12 in (30 cm) chest size—one mother recommended these very highly. Bonnets, hats, mittens, and boots can all be made very successfully from doll-sized patterns, and you will need plenty of these items to keep your baby extra warm.

- Continental or European babywear manufacturers often make baby clothes in smaller sizes than their UK counterparts. These are available in good babywear shops and large stores, but they are expensive. Tiny suits in 50 and 56 cm sizes are wonderful—but they will fit best over disposable nappies rather than terry nappies (a word about nappies below).

- Ordinary brushed cotton baby nighties with tie necks and elasticated wrists can be used with tiny babies. They fit fairly well around the neck and wrists, and look attractive, providing you don't mind if the nightie is twice as long as the baby!

Nappies

How to fit nappies on a premature baby is the most vexed question of all. Ordinary terry-towelling nappies will swamp a tiny baby, weighing under, say, 5½ lbs (2490 g) or 6 lbs (2720 g). Good quality, thick terries are ridiculous.

> I used thin terries folded as small as possible but they still chafed his armpits!

The mothers in our sample all managed to solve the nappy problem in one way or another. Here are some suggestions.

- In hospital, the baby will probably wear special low birth-weight-sized disposable nappies. These gems are just right for the baby, but are not available in shops. We asked leading manufacturers of disposable nappies if they were prepared to market tiny ones to fit babies of around 4 lbs (1814 g) to 5 lbs (2270 g). They were all reluctant to do so, giving their own reasons backed up, they said, by market research. So the 42,000 low birth-weight babies born each year must do without high street disposables. However, you can buy Snugglers in a special 'premature' size from Home Nursing Supplies of Wiltshire (address on page 112). You can only buy them in bulk—packs of either 240 or 120 are available. These premature-sized nappies are not available anywhere else. If you are considering buying prem-sized disposables, see if you can share a pack with another mother.

- If you are considering buying ordinary-sized disposables, a 'mini' size which, although still too big, is better than most. Some mothers bought ordinary disposables and cut them down, fastening them with sellotape!

- The important thing to remember is that your tiny baby will not need high-absorbency nappies for the first couple of months at least. Her bladder is too small to cope with a lot of urine, so her nappies will not be soaking when you change her. So any solution to the 'great nappy problem' is only temporary. When baby is around 6½ lbs (2940 g) she can wear ordinary disposable or terry nappies in comfort. You are therefore looking for a suitable nappy for your baby to wear for the first few months only.

- Many parents used muslin nappies during this time. These are light, thin and soft and eminently suitable. They are available from Mothercare and from nappy manufacturers. Afterwards, when your baby has progressed to ordinary sized nappies, the muslin nappies can still come in useful in many ways—as liners, for example.

- Several mothers bought the cheapest, thinnest nappies available. These could then be folded to fit their small babies. The folding method is called the 'Chinese' or 'Origami' method. Ask your health visitor, midwife or SCBU staff to show you how to do it.

- Shaped nappies can be useful but take longer to dry than ordinary terries. 'Cherub' do packs of twelve shaped nappies, and they are also available from Mothercare. Shaped nappies are a little easier to fit a small baby than folded terries.

- One mother used thin, old nappies, folded all the corners in to make a smaller square, and then folded the nappy as normal.

- Some mothers were advised by a babywear manufacturer to cut ordinary terries in half across the diagonal, and hem the raw edge. This proved difficult as the raw edge is on a bias and therefore awkward to sew properly. However, once achieved, the result was a smaller, triangular-shaped nappy which could be folded again and used. If you did this with say, six terries, you would have a dozen very useful tiny nappies to tide you over the first months. They can be used afterwards, too, in many ways.

- You can make small terry nappies yourself—or get your family and friends to help! Buy terry towelling from a fabric shop and make small squares (try 40 cm). Make sure they are properly hemmed.

- However you solve the 'great nappy problem', you will also have to consider plastic pants. Tiny, low birth-weight plastic pants are available but, be warned that however neatly fitting these pants are, especially around the waist and leg where a good fit is essential, the pants will not fit over a full-sized terry nappy. Make sure you have small enough nappies to fit under these tiny pants. Frilled, lacy, low birth-weight pants are not recommended.

- Several mothers used tie-on plastic pants. With these, you will get an adjustable fit, so that you can use them with any nappies. However, they are still rather large for a tiny baby.

- A sensible suggestion came from one mother. She bought good, long-life pants in the smallest 60 cm size and put a stitch or two in each leg and in the waist. This made sure that the pants fitted snugly to avoid leakage and draughty gaps, and yet there was plenty of room for a bulky nappy. She removed the stitches when her daughter grew older and bigger, and was still using the same pants when her baby was seven months old.

Equipment

Again, remember that your equipment will be the same as that needed for a term baby, with a few small adjustments. A washing-up bowl will do admirably for a bath, and is easier to manage than a baby bath. Your baby needs somewhere warm and cosy to sleep, rather than a big cot. A small carrycot, crib, or lined wicker basket will be suitable. One mother used a wicker washing basket for the first three months! Your sterilizing unit, whether bought or homemade from a plastic container, will be in use not only for bottles but for medicine spoons and droppers. If you are bottle feeding, remember that your baby may need feeding little and often, so more bottles than usual are needed. Have a good supply of bottles and suitable teats.

It is important that your baby comes home to a warm house—or at least, a warm room. Discuss this with your midwife or health visitor. Whatever form of heating you use, it must be safe and capable of heating at least the baby's room to 20 °C (70 °F). Beware of automatic timed heating systems which switch off for certain periods of the day. Premature babies, as we have seen, have immature body temperature regulators, so they find it difficult to keep warm. Your baby will not be discharged until the paediatrician is certain that she can cope with normal room temperatures, but you will still be asked to ensure that the house is warm.

The day of discharge

> The day the three of us came home, I cried. It was a fantastic day.

At last the day arrives when you can take your baby home. You can look forward to resuming normal life, without exhausting trips to the hospital, and you can be a real family. Most parents manage to go together for their baby—it is a special day after all. You will feel excited, happy, relieved, and perhaps a little anxious too. The baby has been cocooned in the security and warmth of the SCBU—will she be able to cope with normal life? The paediatrician will not discharge the baby until he is as sure as he can be that she is *ready* to go home, so you can be confident that the time has come to give your baby a warm, loving home in which to grow up. You may have misgivings

—but this is common in parents with full-term babies too! You are experiencing normal feelings. The best way to make the transition from SCBU to home is to be well-prepared, well-informed about premature babies and about your baby in particular, well-supported by family and friends, and to stay calm, confident, and relaxed.

The actual day of discharge can be rather frustrating. The paediatrician must give your baby a thorough examination and he needs to talk fully with you about the daily care of your baby. However, he also has other duties, some of which may be emergencies or serious cases. Try to be patient if there is a delay.

When your baby has been examined she will be ready to wear her going-home clothes. Make sure you dress her warmly, and wrap her snugly in several warm blankets. Ensure that her head is covered, and that her hands and feet are warm.

The paediatrician or sister will discuss daily care with you. You will probably be asked to make sure the baby is warm, and advice will be given about whether or not to take the baby out for walks in her pram, about visitors, or any other special considerations. This is the time to *ask* about anything you are unsure of—no matter how trivial it may seem.

If your baby is prescribed medicines to take at home, make sure that you know how to administer these. A written set of instructions is useful—it's easy to get confused when two or three separate drugs are prescribed.

Before you go, you will be given clinic appointments. You will be asked to attend the paediatrician's clinic regularly, so that he can check your baby's growth and development. This is to detect early any problems of development or health, so that necessary treatment can begin promptly. The paediatrician can tell if the baby is growing and gaining weight as expected. He may make general examinations of the baby or check up on any relevant problems that caused concern when on SCBU. He can discuss with you any problem or worry you may have. As the baby grows and her muscles develop, developmental assessments can be made.

These give a general indication of her progress, and can help the doctor to detect any potential problems.

Help from the community

Once home, you can begin to care for your baby as though she were an ordinary full-term baby—in fact you may already have been advised to 'treat her normally'. This is good advice *but* with one or two reservations. Your baby is *not* a full-term baby. She was born prematurely, and she will have special needs, particularly in the first months. This is not to say that she is not normal. She is a perfectly normal premature baby—but she may still need a bit of extra care and attention. For the first weeks, she may need frequent, two or three-hourly feeding. She may chill easily. She may be restless, she may need regular medication, and in general she will probably need a bit of extra help to adjust to normal, everyday life. You can be helped in this by a skilled experienced special care community midwife (SCCM). She will already know your baby because she is attached to your local SCBU. She will visit you frequently and can be contacted at all times. She knows a lot about premature babies, and about their daily care. She is experienced in all matters surrounding prematurity and low birth-weight babies. In short, she is a treasured support and source of advice and information. The problem is that in large areas of the United Kingdom these highly trained, invaluable special care community midwives do not exist. Only 15 per cent of our sample had special after-care of this nature. A paediatrician told us that, with premature babies, the follow-up should be extra caring, so that the community team can detect any problems early. Your general practitioner should be extra vigilant too, and parents should receive extra help and support in the early weeks after discharge.

The best supported parents were those who had special care community midwives. Health visitors were on the whole described as kind and morally supportive, but many were somewhat lacking in knowledge and experience of premature babies. It is to be hoped that special care community midwives become more numerous and able to give support to parents in *all* areas of the United Kingdom.

Your family doctor will be aware of the baby's premature arrival and should visit you at home soon after the baby's discharge. He will have her medical history from the SCBU and will already be aware of any problems she has had. A recently trained, enthusiastic general practitioner (GP) will have a considerable fund of knowledge about neonatology and prematurity. An older general practitioner will not be quite so aware of all the facets of prematurity, unless he has attended special courses recently. This is simply because our knowledge about prematurity has grown so rapidly within the last five or ten years. The important thing is to have total confidence in your general practitioner. Try to get to know him. Show that you are *not* neurotic or over-fussy, but that you are genuinely interested in your baby's health and development. Ask for advice and information if you need it. A good general practitioner will encourage you to contact him any time you are worried, at any time of day or night. He *never* minds coming to visit if you are very worried about your baby, and will make a special effort to see you as soon as possible.

The well-baby clinic

When your baby is ready (ask your general practitioner, special care community midwife or health visitor for advice) you can begin to attend your local clinic. This is staffed by health visitors and helpers, and they will be knowledgeable about babies in general. There will also be a doctor in attendance. Ask to see him if you are worried.

At the clinic your baby will have developmental assessments and immunization like any other baby. To do both of these things the clinic staff will count your baby's age from her *due date*, not from her actual birthday. So a baby born in June, but due in August, will have her age counted as *four* months by Christmas, and not as *six* months. The clinic staff will use her corrected age to work out when she needs her first vaccination and to carry out the relevant developmental assessments.

Other sources

Because of the recent, rapid expansion of knowledge about preterm babies, your local community team may not be able to give you the sort of information or advice you are seeking, simply due to the knowledge and experience not yet being widespread. If you need extra advice contact the SCBU, or their local parent support group; the local NCT (National Childbirth Trust) branch; or 'Nippers' national support group (address on page 113).

> It's surprising just how much reassurance a 'prem' mother needs. I found a tremendous amount of comfort talking to parents who had been in the same situation, probably because there are no guidelines to follow with these babies.

Feeding at home

Your baby may still need two or three-hourly feeds, day and night, when she comes home. On the other hand, she may be feeding four-hourly. As feeding is such an individual topic—each baby being unique—we can only give guidelines and suggestions. Talk fully with your special care community midwife, health visitor, or NCT breastfeeding counsellor about any problems that arise.

- Keep your breast pump for a week or two. You may need it for all kinds of situations—expressing when your breasts are engorged, stimulating your supply, expressing to give baby her milk by bottle, especially if you have sore or cracked nipples. Sometimes problems with nipples begin to show up after a few days of full breastfeeding.

- Beware of a drop in your milk supply, due to the baby's feeble suck after the strong stimulation of the pump, or even due to your tension. Use the pump to stimulate your supply between breastfeeds.

- Try not to expect too much from your baby. She needs help and patience to establish a good home feeding routine. Initially, her weight gain may slow down, while she is adjusting herself. Be prepared for this, and discuss feeding fully with your special care community midwife, or health visitor or NCT counsellor.

- Be prepared to be flexible—to give extra bottle feeds if baby gets tired.

Don't forget the supply and demand principle. The more you let your baby suck, the more milk you will produce.

Bottle feeding
Remember you may need extra bottles if baby is feeding two-hourly.

- Remember that the type of formula you use is important. Talk this over with your health visitor if your baby seems discontented.

- The golden rule is to feed little and often—let your baby take as much milk as she can before falling asleep, and feed her frequently, waking her if necessary. A routine is probably a good idea, since many sleepy premature babies cannot be trusted to wake themselves.

Weaning

Your baby is going to need her first solid food at some time or another. Be guided by your health visitor or special care community midwife, but remember that premature babies are a law unto themselves! Look out for the signs that baby needs her first taste of solid food—restlessness, hunger, more frequent feeding, waking at night for a feed after a period of sleeping through, crying. Be prepared for your baby to need solids when *she* indicates her needs. This may be at around the normal *corrected* age of three, four or five months, or it may be earlier. We found that that several mothers of very early babies began giving solid feeds early too—at one or two months *corrected* age. It was quite common for these early babies to want something more solid fairly soon, perhaps when they still weighed only 7 lbs (3175 g) or 8 lbs (3630 g).

> At three months (one month corrected age) my daughter began to show the classic signs of needing solids. My health visitor was dubious, since baby only weighed 7 lbs 4 oz (3290 g). However, she encouraged me to try a little thickened cereal. The result was amazing. The baby loved it, and asked for more. She thrived, and became a lot happier.

It is also common in such cases to find that a mere teaspoon or two of cereal is enough, once or twice a day, for several weeks. It is advisable to avoid wheat products, and to try baby rice, once or twice a day, until the baby shows signs again that she needs more. It is important, however, to take your cue from your *baby*. Start solids when the *baby* is ready.

We have already said that premature babies are different from term babies, during their first few months. They need extra care to become adjusted to normal life. They can be restless, their learning through play is somewhat different and they need extra attention during the first few weeks because of frequent feeds and vulnerability to cold and infection. However, the paediatrician has discharged your baby because she is *ready to begin* to build up her resistance to infection, and to cope with the bustle of normal family life. So take extra care of your baby, be vigilant and spend time with her. The key to success is to avoid *overprotection*. Being extra caring and vigilant is not being overprotective, but preventing your baby from joining in with real family life when she is ready is to deny her the chance to put her prematurity behind her once and for all.

Feeling low

The stress of a premature birth is great, and parents can suffer from the strain for several weeks after baby's discharge, especially if baby is restless and unsettled.

It is important to try to relax, once your baby is home. Admittedly she needs extra care but she is no longer in the SCBU, needing constant medical assessment. This is difficult for some parents to achieve, but others recognize the importance of relaxing in the warmth of the family home, and the consequent benefit for parents and baby.

> I was so accustomed to feeling tense and worried about my baby that it was a good nine months before I began to relax and let go. Immediately, I felt happier, the baby was more content, and suddenly it was good to be alive! I should have relaxed months earlier.

In the early weeks when you are all settling down, establishing a routine and getting to know each other, the best idea is to stay calm, relaxed and loving. Talk things over with your partner, and concentrate on each other as well as on the baby and older children. Forget the decorating that didn't get done, and abandon any great projects. You can take these up again afterwards when you are all settled. By staying close and concentrating on each other, your baby will benefit. She will sense the calmness and she will feel secure. Older children will gradually begin to see that life is back to normal, and you will all be happier, more content, and more stable.

Get practical help from your family and friends, and stay in touch with people who are experienced in the care of premature babies. Some mothers talked with other 'prem' mums, and many were glad of family support. And in the bewildering whirl of these first weeks, keep a sense of proportion—and be prepared to see the funny side!

> There were some moments of light relief—big brother's disbelief when we produced a washing-up bowl to bath baby, and nanny using my precious expressed breast milk to make a cup of tea!

SEVEN

As Your Baby Grows

You will have been advised by the paediatrician to keep the baby warm as she may still have a tendency to lose body heat quickly. This is very important, especially during the early weeks when she is still thin, with little body fat. You will, as time goes on, begin to recognize that she is beginning to stay warm by herself for longer periods. After a month or two, she will not need so much wrapping nor such a hot room. But at first, take care, and ensure that the house—or her room at least—is a constant 20°C (70°F). If heating costs are a problem you may be able to get financial help. Contact the DHSS or your health visitor. In the early days at home make sure that the baby is properly clothed and that her head is covered. A warm bonnet should always be worn—leaving the baby's head bare is just like leaving her chest bare; she would lose a lot of body heat. Hands and feet get cold quickly so soft warm mittens and bootees are advisable. Make sure the baby is warm *before* you put her back in her crib. Blankets will insulate her, and keep her cool, if she goes to bed cool. If she feels a bit cool, cuddle her next to your body in a very warm room, with a warmed blanket or duvet wrapped round both of you. Try feeding her. When she is warm, you can safely put her in the crib. As a guide, four light layers of clothing (vest, stretch suit or nightie, woollen cardigan or fleecy coverall, and shawl) plus bonnet, mitts and bootees—and two warm blankets wrapped round her—should be enough. She needs extra warmth when she sleeps in her crib. One mother put foil under the mattress. Some mothers bought sheepskin or fleecy mattress covers for their baby's crib. Fleece is an ideal insulator, and is used widely in SCBUs to keep tiny babies warm. Suppliers of baby fleeces are listed on page 114.

While we cannot overemphasize the importance of

keeping baby warm, make sure you don't *overheat* her, particularly as she grows older.

Bathing and washing

Don't attempt to bath your baby every day. She only needs a bath every few days. Bath her in a very warm room and have warm towels ready. Keep the bathing operation speedy, dress her quickly, and get her warm.

- A washing-up bowl makes a good bath.

- When changing baby's nappy between feeds, do this quickly in a very warm room. Wash your hands afterwards.

- Keep all the baby equipment clean and dust-free. Wipe down changing mats and surfaces with a solution of Milton. Keep soiled nappies away from the baby, and dispose of them quickly and carefully.

- Baby's skin is delicate. Wipe it gently, and dry carefully.

Visitors and going out

There is no harm in having visitors in the house providing they are not suffering from colds, sore throats, or other ailments. Your baby is prone to infection during the early weeks, so be firm with any runny-nosed visiting children wanting to cuddle your baby! It is important to build up your baby's resistance to germs by exposing her *gradually*, but it is pointless to let her become ill while she is still so tiny. Take steps to prevent infection until she is bigger, but do try to keep a sense of proportion.

Obviously, older children in the family should *not* be prevented from cuddling the new baby—otherwise jealousy and resentment can occur. But if older brothers and sisters have colds or infectious illnesses, try to keep your very small baby away from them, in her pram or crib. However, don't restrain them from touching or cuddling her, or more harm than good will be done. But once baby gets a bit stronger, a good old dose of family germs is no bad thing.

Be guided by your special care community midwife or health visitor as to whether you can take baby out. Much depends on the season, and your baby's weight. There is no harm in taking her out, wrapped warmly, for a few minutes, on a fine, warm day. Your baby will benefit from being outside in the fresh air when she is stronger and bigger.

Remember, above all, to look out for the signs that your baby is ready to join the mainstream of family life. A newly discharged 3½ lb (1580 g) or 4 lb (1814 g) baby needs all the extra protection we have discussed. As she grows older and puts on weight, she will be able to cope with one less blanket, or an hour in the garden, or a gentle tickle session during a nappy change. The trick is to protect, at first, and then gradually step by step aim to give your baby the chance to experience normal baby and childhood.

Gaining weight

Your baby's weight gain will be watched carefully by the special care community midwife or health visitor, who will probably bring scales with her every couple of days at first. It is difficult not to be apprehensive about baby's weight. Remember that the change in routine may cause an initial slowing of weight gain. Weight checks are a good guide to baby's health, and feeding pattern, and can give an early warning of any problems. Use these regular checks to talk fully with her about your baby.

Physical changes

Gradually you will notice changes in your baby. She begins to lay down fat, and therefore begins to look more sturdy, less scrawny and more like a normal baby, with a rounder face, chubby cheeks, fatter arms and legs, and a real bottom! A baby girl's vaginal area will be more fleshy and padded. Her skin will become less fragile, her tummy and chest more in proportion, and her legs and feet less bent. Her umbilical hernia, if she has one, will begin to protrude less. Her hair will begin to grow, and the bald patches on her head begin to disappear, with new hair growth. Eyelashes and eyebrows grow thicker and toenails and fingernails stronger. She will be able to maintain her body temperature more easily. She is growing fast into an ordinary baby, after her extraordinary start in life.

Your welfare clinic, your general practitioner, your health visitor, or your SCBU clinic will be keeping a record of your baby's weight. This is sometimes plotted on a graph to see how she compares with average baby weight patterns.

Your baby will in all probability catch up with her contemporaries, in terms of size and weight, by around her second birthday. It may take longer. But because of recent advances in knowledge about nutritional needs, your baby will have had the best possible start with a carefully structured feeding schedule. This will have given her a better chance than ever before of 'catching up'. Remember to be patient, to give her a good, mixed diet, and to have confidence that she will grow at her own pace.

The restless baby

It is well known that a baby who has spent some time in special care can be fussier and more demanding once at home: 'Low birthweight babies, separated from their mothers, cried more often and were less easily comforted during their first year'.[17]

Although some mothers in our sample reported no difference in this respect, and that their babies were placid and content, there was definitely a tendency for the premature babies in our survey to be restless, demanding and fussy. They needed constant attention and comfort, and cried a great deal.

> When I brought her home I wept. So did she. She was a *most* unhappy baby for four months.

A restless, demanding baby can be hard work—to put it

mildly. And a tired harassed mother can feel worn out, frustrated and angry, short-tempered with her children and partner; altogether life seems unbearable. The solution is to be aware of what is happening, and to be prepared for it, knowing that your baby will settle down eventually. If you 'give in' to your baby, you are *succeeding*, not failing. Pick her up, cuddle her, soothe her, give her a lot of body contact. Even if she does not stop crying straightaway, you are on the right lines. She needs to feel your physical presence. If she is miserable, frustrated and unhappy she will feel better being close to you. Leaving a baby to cry will only exaggerate the situation. You will not spoil her if you pick her up. She *needs* to be near you, to feel your presence. If you satisfy that need, she will be more content and you will have a better, more stable relationship with each other. The whole family will benefit.

Our research revealed several useful tips for dealing with crying, restless babies.

- First and foremost, go through a mental checklist, eliminating reasons one by one. Is she hungry? Thirsty? Warm enough? (even very slight chilling is enough to make a baby discontented and miserable). Is she ill?—has she got a temperature?—off her food? Does she appear to be off colour? (if you think she is, seek medical help). Could she be in pain? Colic is a cause of crying, although it is not as common as is generally thought. Tummyache seems to cause babies a lot of distress, whereas they can easily recover from surgical operations. If nothing is obviously wrong, she may just feel lonely and miserable. Cuddle her, soothe her, carry her around the house, talk softly to her.

- Sit comfortably and calmly in a rocking chair with your baby, rocking gently and rhythmically.

- Try a baby sling. Make sure baby is warmly clothed, and is secure inside the sling. She can hear your heartbeat and feel your warmth. Many mothers recommended baby slings.

- Music can be of great use. Some parents found that music soothed their babies, their tastes ranging from John Denver to Mozart! Or you can buy cassettes of prerecorded sound patterns which are supposed to soothe crying babies. Some are 'womb music', and one electronic gadget we tested sounds like a rhythmical 'shhh' sound. These cassettes and gadgets have proved successful with at least some parents.

- Above all, your baby will want to be near you if she is feeling miserable. Cuddle her, walk round with her, sit with her—and abandon the dirty dishes or wet washing until peace resumes for ten minutes!

- Try feeding her, particularly if you are breastfeeding. The sucking will calm her.

- If you are truly desperate, try a dummy. Make sure it is a small one, because normal ones are too big for premature babies—they tend to gag and spit them out. NUK make dummies in a special shape, available from NCT.

- And remember, it won't last forever!

Medicines

Premature babies are often prescribed medicines. These may include extra vitamins and minerals, and iron. Vitamins may be in the form of drops or tablets. Iron is usually a medicine. All this medication is necessary to boost your baby's low stores of vitamins and minerals, because she missed out on the last few vital weeks in the womb when these stores are laid down.

- These vitamins and minerals may be obtained from your clinic, or you may have a special prescription, to be made up at a pharmacy. Small, independent chemists are more likely to prepare the medication specially for you. Otherwise, ask the SCBU to try to obtain your medication from the hospital pharmacy.

- You will have been shown how to administer the medication, but here are some tips. Crush tablets *well* into very fine powder, not lumps, between two spoons, which should be plastic, so they can be kept in the sterilizer, and *tough*. Ordinary 5 ml clear plastic spoons from the chemist tend to split easily. You can mix all the medicines together, to make a sort of baby cocktail. Use a plastic medicinal measure, as these are translucent and have capacity markings; they look like large thimbles and are obtainable from chemists and hospital pharmacies.

- When the cocktail is ready, give it to your baby a little at a time, using a sterilized plastic spoon. Ensure that the spoon has no sharp edges. The baby should take *all* the medicine.

- If she hates it, and spits it out (babies dislike the taste of the iron medicine) try giving it to her by medicine dropper. These can be bought from your local chemist.

- Another solution is to give the medicine by a bottle and teat, or even by just using an upturned teat. Pour the medicine into the teat a little at a time while the baby is sucking.

- Mothercare do a special inexpensive medicine 'spoon' which looks rather like a long thin tube. It is marked with the capacities in millilitres, and makes medicine giving less troublesome.

- Some parents felt that the iron medicine disagreed with their baby. It was felt that it caused infrequent bowel movements, and that their babies disliked it. However, the iron is *absolutely essential*, so try to keep going. If you experience problems, discuss the matter thoroughly with your paediatrician, general practitioner or special care community midwife.

Common problems

Thrush

The fungus *Candida albicans* is a normal inhabitant of the mouth, intestines and vagina, usually harmless but occasionally causing an infection known as thrush. This appears as white patches in the baby's mouth. Baby can be fretful and restless. Premature babies are extremely susceptible to thrush, so be on the lookout for it. (Some SCBUs give their babies treatment as routine, and the medicine prescribed for the baby on her discharge.) If you suspect thrush your general practitioner, on confirming the diagnosis, will prescribe a suitable medicine which is usually effective, but thrush is stubborn. To prevent reinfection, step up your hygiene precautions, wash your nipples thoroughly if breastfeeding, and ensure that teats are sterile. The baby's bottom may also be affected, since the thrush will be present in her stools. Make sure you have some prescribed cream for her bottom, and that cream is prescribed for nipples if breastfeeding. It is well worth waging total war on thrush, because it makes a baby fretful and may even prevent her from sucking properly.

Colic

Some babies suffer from 'three-month colic'—an odd name since it usually ends by three months—sometimes known as 'evening colic'. The baby starts to cry and behave as though she had a terrible tummyache. The cause is not fully understood. Many parents—of full-term babies too!—tend to name 'colic' as the cause of every crying session, but true colic always displays a definite set of symptoms. Your baby may just be hungry, restless, unsettled, or lonely. Talk with your general practitioner or health visitor to determine whether your baby really is suffering from colic. If she is, a medicine may help, although doctors are reluctant to prescribe medicines for young babies.

A 'sicky' baby

Premature babies are sometimes 'sicky' babies. They bring back milk or food after every feed, with unfailing regularity.

Some parents reported never sitting down to feed a baby without a box of tissues nearby! It is thought that the valve in the stomach, being immature and undeveloped, does not function efficiently, so that food is easily brought back. Happily, the problem is temporary.

A 'snuffly' baby

Premature babies tend to be snuffly and grunty. The tendency is exaggerated by tiny nostrils and airways, and immature muscle control. If your baby is otherwise well, there is no need to be alarmed by her snores and grunts. However, if she has a cold, your general practitioner may prescribe decongestant drops to enable her to breathe more easily.

Puffy eyes and face

Premature babies have a tendency, during the first weeks, to have a high fluid retention level. This often causes a puffiness around her eyes. You may notice this particularly when she has been asleep for a length of time, in one position—one side of her face, and one eye, will look puffy and swollen. This is again normal and temporary. It will gradually disappear. The head and face also seem elongated. Part of the cause is that the baby's head is easily moulded by gravity and atmospheric pressure—after all, she was designed to be in the womb a bit longer, floating in amniotic fluid. A paediatrician assured us that the babies soon grow out of this, and a special care midwife told us that she had noticed a very definite reduction in the incidence of 'premmie' facial characteristics, unlike years ago: 'Babies are growing out of this much earlier now. They are definitely not "prem" looking when I see them at the clinic.'

Teeth

During the last weeks of pregnancy the enamel is forming in the baby's *first* teeth. The enamel on the *second* teeth is formed just after birth. It is therefore possible that a very premature baby may have poor enamel on her first teeth. They may look yellow and patchy. The second teeth may, or may not, be affected. There is a definite link between prematurity and poor tooth enamel. So keep in close contact with a good, conscientious dentist who has a good relationship with children, and who will discuss your baby's teeth fully with you.

As your baby grows a little older her personality will begin to show itself. She will become accustomed to the household noises and family routine. She will grow used to the unfamiliar pattern of day and night, after several weeks in the constant brightness of the SCBU. She will demonstrate her needs clearly. She will begin to wake herself for feeds, to keep herself warm, and to feed quickly and strongly. She will begin to sleep for longer periods, even to sleep through the night (although our survey revealed an average sleeping-through-the-night age of four to six months!). In short, she is leaving her prematurity behind and becoming a normal, typical baby. Give her room to develop, and grow into a happy, healthy child.

Growing up

> A baby who is young and small and has had prolonged RDS is certainly better off going home to a secure, supportive home with competent parents, than if she goes to a stressed family. . . . In fact, in a stimulating and supportive environment this baby will probably be better off than others who were older and healthier at birth but go home to a poor or disorganized family environment.[18]

For many parents, the early months are tinged with anxiety. Will the baby be all right? Will she be normal? After all, she was *so* poorly. . . .

The facts are these. A *very small* minority of low birthweight babies are too handicapped for normal school.[16] Amongst these are the *very few* babies who suffered brain damage either before or just after birth. These babies will need special care, as they grow into childhood and adulthood. However, it is true to say that *your baby's chances of being seriously handicapped are very slim indeed.* If there was any incident during birth or during the neonatal period which gave the paediatrician any cause to suspect brain damage or other handicap, you will have been told. The paediatrician will then be on extra guard to watch the development of your child, to detect early any handicap. This is done at the SCBU clinics. The doctor will watch for persistence of primitive responses, muscular tone and development, and other signs which can indicate that all is not well. If you are worried, stay in contact with your baby's paediatrician. Discuss the matter thoroughly, and express your feelings. In all probability, your worries will be unfounded, but at least your mind will be at rest.

We have established then that the vast majority of premature babies will grow into perfectly healthy, normal children. However, this is often difficult to envisage, especially if you have had no experience of knowing other premature babies. Most of the parents in our survey were encouraged by the 'before and after' photographs of SCBU babies, or by talking with other 'prem' parents.

> He is now a lively, chatty 3½ year old, quite up with his own age group in all respects.

> She is now the tallest in her class—the brightest and most beautiful.

Will she be a bit slow at school?

It used to be the case that premature babies subsequently had problems with learning. This is no longer held to be valid. Medical knowledge has advanced so far and so rapidly that today's premature infants not only have a better chance than ever of surviving, but also they have the benefit of this tremendous knowledge about brain development, nutrition, metabolic requirements and preventive measures. Early research showed that 40 per cent of babies born prematurely subsequently had intellectual problems. Research done in the early 1970s showed that this had dropped to nearer 5 per cent! And comparing *these* results with studies done in the last two years shows that recent survivors of respiratory distress syndrome are obtaining more optimal developmental scores. So the belief that developmental impairment is a common characteristic of babies born prematurely is nonsense. *Your baby will, in all probability, grow up to be the sort of child she would have been anyway.*

> The rate of development is generally unaffected by premature birth. The rate of development seems to depend on underlying maturational processes that are progressing on a preset schedule, that continues to unfold whether the infant is in the womb or an incubator.[19]

Your baby's development

We have said, quite firmly and categorically, that your baby's prematurity has little to do with her eventual intellectual ability. However, premature babies have a *normal* track of development during the early years which is different from full-term babies. You should not expect your premature baby to behave like a full-term baby during her first year or so. She probably won't. She will have her own characteristics which are typical of premature babies. After the first year or so, these special characteristics fade, and your baby will behave more and more like her contemporary, full-term friends. By the time she is at playgroup—and certainly by the time she is at school—she will be indistinguishable from her full-term peers. She will be the child she was meant to be—gifted or average, musical or creative, athletic or contemplative.

If we were to draw a graph, plotting the development of premature babies compared with their full-term peers, in terms of physical factors like weight or height, or skills like vocabulary size, or motor coordination, we would find that premature babies lag behind for a while, and 'catch up' eventually. In other words, she will get there later.

It is important to say here that premature babies are not all alike. There is a vast difference between a seriously ill 25-week baby, weighing 1 lb (450 g) with many complications and setbacks, and perhaps only discharged from SCBU at five months of age weighing 5 lbs (2260 g), and a 35-week baby, weighing 5 lbs (2260 g) at birth and suffering only from a little immaturity. And of course there are many cases in between. Naturally we must expect the very tiny baby to take longer to 'catch up' and the older baby may perhaps show no real lag.

Barbara DiVitto and Susan Goldberg in their book[20] stress the importance of taking baby's age from the *post-term*, instead of *postnatal* date. For the first year, or longer if baby is very premature, you would count her age from the date she *should* have been born.

The whole question of the developmental milestones causes more bother than almost anything else, amongst parents of full-term babies as well as premature babies! Many parents in our survey had something to say about these elusive milestones, especially when their babies were showing the typical preterm characteristic of an initial lag.

Most of the parents who wrote to us felt that the first few weeks especially were rather anxious ones in this respect. Waiting for the first smile seems to go on for ever. Remember to take the baby's age from her due date, not her birth date. She will probably smile at a *corrected* age of six weeks (like full-term babies) although some smile earlier because of all the extra stimulation from parents. Incidentally, it is known that premature babies display much more 'reflex' smiling than full-term infants, though the reason for this is not known. This sort of smile is not in response to you but is a sort of uncontrolled flicker of a smile disappearing as suddenly as it came, apparently for no reason. This is not a 'true' smile, which is a deliberate act, more than likely displaying pleasure upon seeing her parents.

> It bothered me not to know *when* to expect him to do things, such as when he would respond to things like mobiles, faces etc. I wanted to be ready with the stimulation when *he* was ready for it, and no-one seemed able to tell me just when to expect such things.

The answer is that your baby *will* respond when she is ready. If you become distracted with worry, talk to your general practitioner, but you should be aware that premature babies *do* show an initial lack of response and are slow at first to display developmental stages. She is too busy growing, gaining strength, and maturing! Give her a chance, be patient and watchful, and remember that she *will* do everything, but in her own time.

Your baby will 'catch up' with her contemporaries by the age of two if not before, but you should be aware that, besides showing a lag, premature babies differ in many respects from full-term babies in their *early* development. Most of these differences disappear by the first birthday.

The rate of motor-skill development is affected, particularly those skills which are normally achieved between six and twelve months.

Premature babies also 'play' differently. The way they handle and explore objects and toys is different. Barbara DiVitto and Susan Goldberg[21] describe research which shows that premature babies with a history of respiratory problems tend to explore toys less with their mouths, and that premature babies do fewer 'combined' activities, such as putting bricks into a container. They are more likely to play with the brick *or* the box but not to explore the possibility of the box as a container for the bricks. Premature babies are less actively involved in exploring objects thoroughly. They are more easily distracted. Manipulative skills of course are delayed. There is also evidence to suggest that premature infants seem to be inefficient information processors. They are not good at understanding or realizing the significance of the stimulus presented to them. Parents engaged in play with their babies often notice that their efforts to stimulate are ignored or rejected. It is thought that premature babies *do* need stimulation but that they easily become overloaded and unable to cope. We have seen that babies feed better in the early days when the mother does not attempt any social interaction. It is suggested that *small* amounts of information or stimulus, presented to the baby *regularly* at a slow rate, is the best way to achieve optimal development.

All parents should be aware that the biggest single factor affecting a child's development and achievement is the home environment. This is such a well-known concrete fact amongst child care and education experts that it is a wonder more parents do not recognize it. It is all the more important for parents of premature babies to remember that the quality of the baby's home environment will have a direct, permanent effect on her development. A good home environment has little to do with luxury accommodation, the number of electronic gadgets, or two cars in the garage. It does not matter whether a child has one parent or two, expensive toys or homemade ones, designer clothes or hand-me-downs. What *does* matter is your relationship with your child.

> In a study which attempted to predict the developmental ability of preterm infants, lots of assessments were used, e.g. obstetric history, paediatric examinations, visual-attention tasks, infant development tests, and home visits. It was found that the assessments of the home environment and the quality of the parent–child relationship, were better predictors than information about birth, delivery, or other early medical events.[22]

To give your child the best chance of achieving her optimum personal attainment level, you should know her thoroughly, understand her needs, support, stimulate and encourage her at every stage, from her earliest weeks to young adulthood, and particularly during her first five years. Avoid overstimulation, during the first twelve months, especially. In the early weeks she will need your physical contact and warmth. Watch her development. *She* will give *you* cues to tell you when to encourage her to sit up, to build brick towers, to stand, to walk, to draw, to do jigsaws. Try not to compare her with others. Instead, be aware of the normal, developmental sequence of babies and children. If you are not familiar with the 'milestones', such as when babies first crawl, walk, etc., we recommend that you buy a good book (see page 76), or talk fully with your health visitor or general practitioner. Armed with this knowledge, you have a good guide as to what your baby will do next. By using her corrected age for the first year or so you will have a better idea of her stage of development, but remember to follow *her* cues first. For instance, you may notice that her visual attention is caught by a particular colour of dress you are wearing. You know then to introduce bright mobiles, and friezes on her bedroom wall. If she listens intently to a sound somewhere in the room, introduce her to soft music, or a tinkling toy, or a rattle. Try to capitalize on what she can do, by giving her more of the same. If she begins to grasp your fingers, give her toys to hold for a moment. If she begins to pull herself upright using your hands, make a game of it and let her enjoy it.

Remember to give her new information or experiences in small doses, but regularly. Don't try to do too much, she will 'switch off' or cry. Practice will tell you how much she can cope with at one time. Follow her cues, and be ready with the stimulation. Together as a loving family, you can come through the difficult days, and grow together, learning from each other, giving your baby the best possible chance of developing into a healthy happy child. And whether she was born prematurely or not will no longer matter.

Medical Glossary

This is not meant to be a definitive list, but is rather a guide to the more common terms encountered by parents.

Anaemia too few red blood cells to carry oxygen
Anoxia a period without oxygen
Antibiotics drugs used to combat infection
Apnoea a period without breathing
Aspiration inhalation of fluid into the lungs, such as milk, meconium
Atresia absence of a natural opening; usually operable

Bilirubin yellow pigment from red blood cell breakdown; causes jaundice
Blood gases test on a blood sample from baby to show oxygen and carbon dioxide levels
Bradycardia slowing of the heart rate
Brain scan an ultrasound scan of the brain to show the inner structures
Bronchopulmonary dysplasia hardening of parts of the lung tissues; associated with long oxygen therapy

Caput normal, slight swelling on the head present at birth, caused by pressure
Cardiograph tracing of the heart beat
Cephalhaematoma swelling on the head, develops after birth; lasts several weeks but will subside; often on one side of the head only
Cerebral haemorrhage bleeding in the brain
Chest drain small tube put into chest when lung has collapsed, to help reinflate it
CPAP continuous positive airways pressure
Cyanosis reduced level of oxygen causes this condition where skin, lips and nails become a bluish colour

Endotracheal tube plastic tube inserted through mouth and down to main lung passage, used to assist breathing in CPAP or ventilation

Exchange transfusion blood transfusion given to ill babies with jaundice; exchanges the toxic blood for fresh donor blood

Haemoglobin iron content of red blood cells that carries oxygen

Hernia occurs when internal organs protrude through the structures that cover them

HMD hyaline membrane disease, a lung problem causing difficulty with breathing

Hydrocephaly an excess of 'water in the brain', causing enlargement of the head

Hyper too high

Hypo too low

Hypocalcaemia a low level of calcium in the blood

Hypoglycaemia a low blood sugar level. Premature babies are screened regularly initially—four to eight hourly, by a blood sample dropped onto a special preprepared plastic stick, a Dextrostix; treatment is giving a dextrose solution or a feed

Hypothermia an abnormally low temperature, below 35 °C

Infusion a drip to give fluids into the body

Inhalation the breathing in of air, vapour or other substances into the lungs

Inguinal hernia inguinal—area in the groin; hernia protrudes through inguinal muscles and causes swelling in the groin; commonest in boys, and treated by surgery at a later date

IPPV intermittent positive pressure ventilation; ventilating the baby's lungs mechanically to breathe for the baby

IVH intraventricular haemorrhage bleeding within the ventricles of the brain from small blood vessels

Meconium baby's first motion, a greeny-black sticky substance

Meconium aspiration inhalation at birth of meconium into the lungs; a serious condition which needs special care and treatment

Meningitis infection in the tissues surrounding the brain and spine

Microcephaly a small head

Moulding the change in shape of the baby's head caused at birth by pressure from the mother's birth canal; the soft skull bones easily allow for this; moulding resolves itself

Necrotizing enterocolitis (NEC) inflammation of a section of the wall of the intestines; the baby is very ill with severe diarrhoea and blood in the motions; surgery is usually the treatment

NG feeds Nasogastric feeds, given by a tube which passes down the nose into the stomach

Oedema swelling in the tissues under the skin, due to excess fluid

PDA patent ductus arteriosus—the temporary flap in the heart remains open causing the baby to have a heart murmur

Physiotherapy chest physiotherapy, vibration to the chest wall by hands or a small electric toothbrush to loosen mucus in the lungs; suctioning away the mucus from the airways follows

Pneumonia inflammation of the lungs due to an infection or irritation following aspiration, such as meconium aspiration or milk inhalation

Pneumothorax air between the chest wall and lung caused by an air leak from the lung; causes the lung to collapse

Retrolentalfibroplasia blindness caused by unnecessarily giving high oxygen levels; blood vessels behind the eye burst and cause blindness; rarely occurs now due to careful monitoring and better understanding of giving oxygen

Sepsis the presence of infection

Spina bifida a condition in which the spine has developed abnormally, the spinal cord can protrude through; occurs in varying degrees of severity

Top-up transfusion a small blood transfusion to treat anaemia

Umbilical area area of the navel
Umbilical hernia protrusion of some of the intestines at the umbilical area.

Notes

1 DHSS statistics for 1982 (Low weight birth and mortality—Notification').
2 All figures taken from (a) *British Journal of Obstetrics and Gynaecology*, 89, 887–891, 1982; (b) *British Journal of Hospital Medicine*, 28, 455–461, 1982; *British Medical Journal*, 286, 454–457, 1983.
3 Figures taken from DHSS statistics. The DHSS do not yet keep statistics for survival by gestational age.
4 Susan Goldberg and Barbara A. DiVitto, *Born Too Soon: Preterm Birth and Early Development*, W. H. Freeman and Co., 1983.
5 See Priscilla Alderson, *Special Care for Babies in Hospital*, booklet from National Association for the Welfare of Children in Hospital, 1983.
6 Goldberg and DiVitto, op. cit.
7 Alderson, op. cit.
8 Ibid.
9 'Survey into Special Care Units', NAWCH, 1983.
10 Alderson, op. cit.
11 S. Scott and M. Richards, 'Nursing low-birthweight babies on lambswool', *Lancet*, 12 May, 1979.
12 'Survey into Special Care Units', NAWCH, 1983.
13 E. Helsing and F. Savage King, *Breast Feeding in Practice*, Oxford University Press, 1982.
14 Ibid.
15 *Expressing and Storing Breast Milk* and *Breastfeeding if Your Baby Needs Special Care*.
16 Goldberg and DiVitto, op. cit.
17 Alderson, op. cit.
18 Goldberg and DiVitto, op. cit.
19 Ibid.
20 Ibid.
21 Ibid.
22 Ibid.

Further Reading

Department of Employment, *Employment Rights for the Expectant Mother*, booklet, 1982.

E. Friedrich and Cherry Rowland, *The Twins Handbook*, Robson Books Ltd., 1983.

La Lèche League, *Beginning Breastfeeding*, leaflet.

La Lèche League, *Breastfeeding your Premature Baby*, pamphlet revised September 1984.

Penelope Leach, *Baby and Child*, Penguin, 1977.

Maternity Alliance, *Money for Mothers and Babies*, leaflet.

Maire Messenger, *The Breastfeeding Book*, Century Publishing, 1982.

B. Nash (ed.), *The Complete Book of Babycare—From Conception to 3 Years*, Octopus Ltd. for Marks and Spencer, 1980.

National Association for the Welfare of Children in Hospital, *Your Baby in Special Care: Notes for Parents*, leaflet.

National Childbirth Trust, *Thinking about Breastfeeding*, leaflet.

Useful Addresses

Anthony Bayles (baby fleeces)
Prospect Road
Alresford
Hampshire SO24 9QF (096273 3025)

The Association for Post-Natal Illness
7 Gowan Avenue
Fulham
London SW6

The Association of Breastfeeding Mothers (newsletters and counsellors)
c/o Peggy Thomas (Secretary)
131 Mayow Road
London SE26

Babygro Ltd. (low birth weight clothes)
16 Berkeley Street
London W1X 6AP (01 629 5834)

BLISS (a charity which raises money to buy SCBU equipment and to train doctors in neonatal care)
Baby Life Support Systems
c/o Josie Evans (Secretary)
298 Woodlands Avenue
Eastcote
Ruislip
Middlesex HA4 9QZ

Claire Harding (low birth weight baby clothes)
42 Durham Road
Wilpshire
nr. Blackburn
Lancs.

Compassionate Friends (for bereaved parents)
5 Lower Clifton Hill
Clifton
Bristol BS8 1BT

Direct Diagnostics Ltd. (electronic soother)
6A High Street
Crawley
Sussex RH10 1BJ

Dollycare (Cosby) Ltd. (low birth weight clothes)
13 Elm Tree Road
Cosby
Leicester LE9 5SR (0533 773013)

Foresight (Pre-conceptual Care Group)
Woodhurst
Hydestile
Godalming
Surrey GU8 4AY

Harringtons Ltd. (low birth weight clothes)
83 High Street
Westerham
Kent

Home Nursing Supplies (premature-size disposable nappies)
Headquarters Road
West Wilts Trading Estate
Westbury
Wiltshire BA13 4JJ (Westbury (0373) 822313)

Jaygee Cassettes (baby soother tape)
The Baby Soother
12 Broderip
Cossington
Bridgwater
Somerset (0278 722637)

Joan Custance (low birth weight baby clothes and nappies)
119 Slyne Road
Bolton-le-Sands
via Carnforth
Lancs. LA5 8AJ

La Lèche League (Great Britain) Ltd.
BM 3424
London WC1V 6XX (01 404 5011)

Maternity Alliance (information on mothers' rights)
309 Kentish Town Road
London NW5 2TJ (01 267 7477)

National Association for the Welfare of Children in Hospital (NAWCH)
7 Exton Street
London SE1 8UE (01 261 1738)

National Childbirth Trust (NCT)
9 Queensborough Terrace
London W2 3TB (01 221 3833)

Nippers, a National Support Group for Parents of Special Care Babies
c/o St. Mary's Hospital
Praed Street
London

Poppets (clothes for premature babies)
Stephanie Roberts
24 Hollin Lane
Leeds 16

The Pre-Eclamptic Toxaemia Society
c/o Dawn James
88 Plumberow
Lee Chapel North
Basildon
Essex

Robbins Medical Supplies Ltd. (Robbins Nurser Breast Pump)
22 The Avenue
Hitchin
Herts. SG4 9RL

The Stillbirth and Perinatal Death Association
37 Christchurch Hill
London NW3 1LA

Tiddleywinks (low birth weight clothes)
7 Banks Avenue
Golcar
Huddersfield HD7 4LZ (0484 656031)

The Twins Club
27 Woodham Park Road
Woodham
Weybridge
Surrey

Winganna Products (baby fleeces)
Sandy Hill Cottage
Sandy Haven
St Ishmaels
Haverfordwest
Dyfed SA62 3DL

Weight Conversion Chart

Grams	lbs	ozs	Grams	lbs	ozs
700	1	8½	2000	4	6½
750	1	10½	2050	4	8½
800	1	12	2100	4	10
850	1	14	2150	4	11¾
900	1	15½	2200	4	13½
950	2	1½	2250	4	15¼
1000	2	3¼	2300	5	1
1050	2	5	2350	5	3
1100	2	6¾	2400	5	4½
1150	2	8½	2450	5	6½
1200	2	10½	2500	5	8¼
1250	2	12½	2550	5	10
1300	2	14	2600	5	11¾
1350	2	15¾	2650	5	13½
1400	3	1½	2700	5	15¼
1450	3	3¼	2750	6	1
1500	3	5	2800	6	2¾
1550	3	6¾	2850	6	4½
1600	3	8½	2900	6	6¼
1650	3	10¼	2950	6	8
1700	3	12	3000	6	9¾
1750	3	13¾	3050	6	11½
1800	3	15½	3100	6	13¼
1850	4	1¼	3150	6	15
1900	4	3	3200	7	0¾
1950	4	4¾	3250	7	2¾

Index